Visit our website

to find out about other books from Churchill Livingstone
and our sister companies in Harcourt Health Sciences

Register free at
www.harcourt-international.com

and you will get

- the latest information on new books, journals and electronic products in your chosen subject areas

- the choice of e-mail or post alerts or both, when there are any new books in your chosen areas

- news of special offers and promotions

- information about products from all Harcourt Health Sciences companies including W. B. Saunders, Churchill Livingstone, and Mosby

You will also find an easily searchable catalogue, online ordering, information on our extensive list of journals...and much more!

Visit the Harcourt Health Sciences website today!

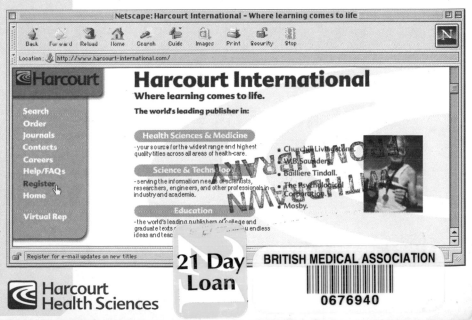

MCQ Companion to
General and Systematic Pathology

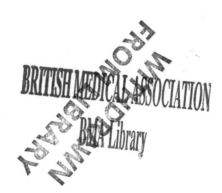

Publisher: Timothy Horne
Project Editor: Michele Staunton
Production Controller: Nancy Arnott
Designer: Erik Bigland

MCQ Companion to General and Systematic Pathology

Simon S. Cross BSc MB BS MD FRCPath
Senior Lecturer and Honorary Consultant, University of Sheffield Medical School and Central Sheffield University Hospitals Trust, Sheffield

THIRD EDITION

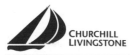
CHURCHILL
LIVINGSTONE

EDINBURGH LONDON NEW YORK PHILADELPHIA ST LOUIS SYDNEY TORONTO 2000

CHURCHILL LIVINGSTONE
An imprint of Harcourt Publishers Limited

© Harcourt Publishers Limited 2000

 is a registered trademark of Harcourt Publishers Limited

The right of Simon S. Cross to be identified as author of this
work has been asserted by him in accordance with the
Copyright, Designs and Patents Act 1988

First edition 1992
Second edition 1996
Third edition 2000

ISBN 0-443-06482-2

British Library Cataloguing in Publication Data
A catalogue record for this book is available from the British
Library

Library of Congress Cataloging in Publication Data
A catalog record for this book is available from the Library of
Congress

Note
Medical knowledge is constantly changing. As new information
becomes available, changes in treatment, procedures, equipment
and the use of drugs become necessary. The author and the
publishers have taken care to ensure that the information given
in this text is accurate and up to date. However, readers are
strongly advised to confirm that the information, especially with
regard to drug usage, complies with the latest legislation and
standards of practice.

The
publisher's
policy is to use
paper manufactured
from sustainable forests

Typeset by IHM(Cartrif), Loanhead, Scotland
Printed by Bell & Bain Ltd., Glasgow

How to use this book

Although recently there have been changes in medical education towards more investigative learning and assessment, multiple-choice examinations still form a staple part of student assessment at most schools. Multiple-choice questions are marked objectively (and usually rapidly by machine) and they can cover a large body of knowledge in a relatively short time. The disadvantage of them is that they are a 'closed' system of questioning which does not allow additional ideas or information to be expressed.

This book is a collection of 320 multiple-choice questions that are divided into subject chapters corresponding with those in *General and Systematic Pathology*, 3rd edition (Churchill Livingstone, 2000), edited by Professor J.C.E. Underwood. Full explanatory answers are given for all the questions so that this book may be used as a useful complement to the main textbook or to any other pathology textbook. All the questions take the form of a stem with five branches which must be marked 'true' or 'false'. This is the most commonly used system of questioning in British medical schools and is usually scored as +1 for a correct response, −1 for an incorrect response and 0 for no response.

A book like this can be used in several ways to assist learning and preparation for examinations. A topic in pathology, such as cardiovascular pathology, could be studied in a textbook and then appropriate questions used to consolidate that knowledge. When preparing for examinations students may wish to practise answering a mixed collection of questions. This book does not include a chapter of mixed questions but such a variety could be achieved by answering, for example, the first question in each chapter. There are variations between medical schools in the timing of pathology teaching and whether other subjects are examined concurrently, so it is not possible to make definitive recommendations about a satisfactory level of achievement on these questions; however, a mark of above 60% (using the marking scheme given above) would probably be adequate.

Sheffield, 2000
S.S.C.

Acknowledgements

I must thank the medical undergraduates I have taught in Cardiff and Sheffield for using the questions as part of their tutorial teaching and making helpful comments on them. Andy Bull, Angus Molyneux and Claire Whitehead have worked their way through all the questions of the first edition, and I thank them for their useful suggestions. Any errors that remain are of course entirely my responsibility but I hope that rigorous checking will have eliminated the majority of them.

Contents

1

Introduction to pathology

1.1 **The following pathology subspecialties are correctly defined:**
- **A.** Haematology — the study of infectious diseases.
- **B.** Toxicology — the study of abnormal chromosomes or genes.
- **C.** Immunology — the study of the specific defence mechanisms in the body.
- **D.** Forensic pathology — the application of pathology to legal purposes.
- **E.** Histopathology — the diagnosis of disease by examining tissues.

1.2 **The following cellular components and functions are correctly associated:**
- **A.** Nucleus — oxidative metabolism.
- **B.** Lysosomes — enzymic degradation.
- **C.** Cell membrane — functional envelope of the cell.
- **D.** Nucleus — genes encoded in DNA.
- **E.** Mitochondria — immune recognition.

1.3 **Health screening programmes:**
- **A.** Always use pathological examination of body cells as the primary screening modality.
- **B.** Have a better take up in lower rather than higher socioeconomic classes.
- **C.** Can be devised without knowledge of the pathology of a disease.
- **D.** Exist in most developed countries for carcinoma of the uterine cervix.
- **E.** Exist in most developed countries for carcinoma of the lung.

1.1   **A.   False.**   Haematology is the study of disorders of blood. Microbiology is the study of infectious diseases and the organisms responsible for them.

B.   False.   Toxicology is the study of the effects of known or suspected poisons. The study of abnormal chromosomes and genes is called genetics.

C.   True.

D.   True.

E.   True.

1.2   **A.   False.**   Oxidative metabolism occurs in the mitochondria.

B.   True.

C.   True.

D.   True.

E.   False.   HLA substances are responsible for immune recognition.

1.3   **A.   False.**   In cervical screening cells scraped from the cervix are examined cytologically but in many other screening programmes, such as that for breast cancer, other primary modalities, such as radiography, are used.

B.   False.   A problem with most screening programmes is adequate coverage of the population at risk of the disease; in most countries those classified as being in the lower socioeconomic classes have a much lower attendance rate than middle and upper socioeconomic classes.

C.   False.   Detailed knowledge of the pathology of a disease is required to plan the optimal screening modality and screening interval.

D.   True.

E.   False.   Although lung carcinomas may be visible on chest radiographs this usually occurs late in the disease and no satisfactory primary screening modality for lung carcinoma has yet been devised.

2

Characteristics, classification and incidence of disease

2.1 **The following prefixes and suffixes are correctly defined:**
- **A.** Hypo — a deficiency below normal.
- **B.** Meta — an excess over normal.
- **C.** Itis — an inflammatory process.
- **D.** Plasia — a disorder of growth.
- **E.** Oma — a tumour.

2.2 **These definitions are correct:**
- **A.** Prognosis — the incidence and distribution of a disease.
- **B.** Pathogenesis — the cause of a disease.
- **C.** Aetiology — the mechanism by which a disease is caused.
- **D.** Sequelae — the complications of a disease.
- **E.** Idiopathic — without a known cause.

2.3 **The following changes in disease patterns have occurred in Europe and North America in the past 50 years:**
- **A.** The death rate from lung cancer has fallen in females.
- **B.** The death rate from road accidents has fallen since 1970.
- **C.** The death rate from suicide has fallen.
- **D.** The death rates from strokes (cerebrovascular accidents) have risen.
- **E.** The death rate from heart ischaemia has risen.

(Answers overleaf)

2.1 **A.** **True.** Examples are hypoglycaemia (low blood sugar) and hypothyroidism (lack of functional activity of the thyroid gland).
B. **False.** Hyper- is an excess over normal, meta- denotes a change from one state to another (e.g. metaplasia).
C. **True.** Examples include appendicitis, cholecystitis and colitis.
D. **True.** Hypoplasia is a lack of growth, and hyperplasia an excess of growth.
E. **True.** All tumours have -oma as their suffix: carcinoma, melanoma, lymphoma, sarcoma.

2.2 **A.** **False.** The prognosis of a disease is its expected outcome.
B. **False.** Pathogenesis is the mechanism by which a disease is caused; the aetiology is the cause of the disease.
C. **False.**
D. **True.**
E. **True.** Other terms for diseases without a known cause include primary, essential, spontaneous and cryptogenic.

2.3 **A.** **False.** The death rate from lung cancer in females has shown a steep rise since 1955 with no decline in the rate of increase. In males the death rate from lung cancer peaked in the mid 1980s and has shown a slight fall since then.
B. **True.**
C. **False.** The suicide rate in all countries falls during wartime and was low in the early 1950s. Since then it has shown a steady increase in both sexes.
D. **False.** The death rate from strokes has fallen slightly in both sexes since 1950 in Europe and North America. This may be related to better control of blood pressure by drugs.
E. **False.** Although ischaemic heart disease is very common in Europe and North America the death rates from it have fallen in both sexes since 1950.

3

Genetic and environmental causes of disease

3.1   Class II HLA antigens:
   A. Are expressed on the surface of all nucleated cells.
   B. Are coded by alleles found at loci labelled A, B and C.
   C. Are involved in the initiation of immune responses.
   D. Enable cytotoxic T-lymphocytes to eliminate virus-infected cells.
   E. Reside on human chromosome 6.

3.2   The following HLA antigens and diseases have significant positive associations:
   A. B27 — ankylosing spondylitis.
   B. DR5 — rheumatoid disease.
   C. DR4 — Hashimoto's thyroiditis.
   D. DR3 — coeliac disease.
   E. DR3 — insulin-dependent diabetes mellitus.

3.3   Human *pax* genes:
   A. Are analogous with the homeobox genes in the *Drosophila* fruitfly.
   B. Play a major role in embryogenesis.
   C. Have an entirely maternal inheritance.
   D. Lie on DNA outside the cell nucleus.
   E. Are defective in familial mitochondrial encephalopathy.

3.4   The following are X-linked genetic disorders:
   A. Glucose-6-phosphate dehydrogenase deficiency.
   B. Duchenne muscular dystrophy.
   C. Patau's syndrome.
   D. Neurofibromatosis.
   E. Ataxia telangiectasia.

(Answers overleaf)

3.1   **A.** **False.**   Class I antigens are expressed on all nucleated cells. Class II antigens are expressed on antigen-presenting cells (such as Langerhans' cells).
   B. **False.**   Class II antigens are coded for by alleles at DP, DQ and DR. Class I antigens are coded by genes at loci A, B and C.
   C. **True.**   Class II antigens are involved in the initiation of immune responses.
   D. **True.**
   E. **True.**

3.2   **A.** **True.**
   B. **False.**   DR4 is associated with rheumatoid disease.
   C. **False.**   DR5 is associated with Hashimoto's disease.
   D. **True.**
   E. **True.**

3.3   **A.** **True.**
   B. **True.**   If the analogous genes in mice (*hox* genes) are defective they can produce a congenital malformation resembling spina bifida.
   C. **False.**   *Pax* genes are inherited in the usual way from paternal and maternal DNA. Mitochondrial DNA has an entirely maternal inheritance.
   D. **False.**   *Pax* genes lie in nuclear DNA. The only human DNA which lies outside the nucleus is in mitochondria.
   E. **False.**   Familial mitochondrial encephalopathy is due to a defective mitochondrial gene.

3.4   **A.** **True.**
   B. **True.**
   C. **False.**   Patau's syndrome is characterised by trisomy of chromosome 13.
   D. **False.**   Neurofibromatosis is a single gene autosomal disorder.
   E. **False.**   Ataxia telangiectasia is due to an excessive fragility of chromosomes.

3.5   The following diseases are caused by fungi:

    A. Onchocerciasis.

    B. Aspergillosis.

    C. Malaria.

    D. Toxoplasmosis.

    E. Cryptococcosis.

3.6   The human major histocompatibility complex (MHC):

    A. Resides on chromosome 11.

    B. Is composed of human leukocyte antigen (HLA) genes.

    C. Codes for three classes of antigens.

    D. Will be identical in dizygotic twins.

    E. Codes for blood group antigens.

3.7   The following diseases are caused by exotoxins released from bacteria:

    A. Pseudomembranous colitis.

    B. Botulism.

    C. Scalded skin syndrome.

    D. Cholera.

    E. Diphtheria.

3.8   The following diseases are caused by bacteria:

    A. Toxic shock syndrome.

    B. Syphilis.

    C. Infectious mononucleosis.

    D. Rubella.

    E. Rabies.

(Answers overleaf)

3.5 **A. False.** Onchocerciasis is caused by *Onchocerca volvulus*, a microfilarial roundworm.
  B. True. *Aspergillus* species may cause various diseases in humans, including allergic asthma, mycetoma and invasive aspergillosis.
  C. False. Malaria is caused by the *Plasmodium* group of protozoa.
  D. False. *Toxoplasma gondii* is another protozoan.
  E. True. *Cryptococcus neoformans* is a yeast-like fungus which causes systemic infection in immunosuppressed humans.

3.6 **A. False.** The human MHC is situated on chromosome 6.
  B. True. There are six pairs of allelic genes (A, B, C, DP, DQ, DR).
  C. False. There are two classes of HLA antigens. Class I antigens are expressed on the surface of all nucleated cells; class II antigens are expressed on the surface of cells such as antigen-presenting macrophages which react with T-lymphocytes.
  D. False. The human MHC will be identical only in monozygotic twins.
  E. False.

3.7 **A. True.** *Clostridium difficile* produces the toxin which causes pseudomembranous colitis.
  B. True. Botulism is caused by ingestion of an exotoxin produced by *Clostridium botulinum*.
  C. True. The syndrome is caused by an exotoxin produced by *Staphylococcus pyogenes*.
  D. True. Cholera is caused by the enterotoxin produced by *Vibrio cholerae*.
  E. True. *Corynebacterium diphtheriae* makes an exotoxin which causes a neuropathy and cardiomyopathy.

3.8 **A. True.** This syndrome is caused by an exotoxin which is produced by *Staphylococcus aureus*.
  B. True. Syphilis is caused by the spirochaete *Treponema pallidum*.
  C. False. Infectious mononucleosis is caused by infection with the Epstein–Barr virus.
  D. False. Rubella is caused by a togavirus.
  E. False. Rabies is caused by a rhabdovirus.

4

Diagnostic pathology in clinical practice

4.1 Exfoliative cytology:

A. Involves the study of wax-embedded pieces of tissue.
B. Is performed on cells aspirated through a fine needle.
C. Is used to screen for carcinoma of the uterine cervix.
D. May be used to diagnose carcinoma of the bronchus.
E. Is often used in the diagnosis of breast lesions.

4.2 In-situ hybridisation (ISH):

A. Detects proteins on the surfaces of cells.
B. Can be used to detect Epstein–Barr virus in tissue sections.
C. Can only be visualised by radioisotopic methods.
D. Uses specifically-raised monoclonal antibodies.
E. Can be used to detect specific mRNA in cells.

(Answers overleaf)

4.1 **A. False.** Cytology is the examination of dispersed cells rather than pieces of tissue.

B. False. Exfoliative cytology examines cells which have been shed or scraped from an epithelial surface. Fine-needle aspiration cytology is useful for organs which do not have easily accessible epithelial surfaces.

C. True. The main use of exfoliative cytology in Britain is in the national screening programme for cervical carcinoma. Cells are scraped from the cervix with a spatula and then smeared on slides before staining and cytological examination.

D. True. Brushings of bronchial mucosa can produce a good yield of cells which may allow the diagnosis of carcinoma to be made.

E. False. The cytological diagnosis of breast lesions is usually made on samples obtained by fine-needle aspiration. Cytology of shed cells in nipple discharge has not proved very useful.

4.2 **A. False.** Immunohistochemistry is used to detect proteins on the surfaces of cells. ISH detects DNA or mRNA within the cell nucleus and cytoplasm.

B. True. One of the more common diagnostic uses of ISH is detection of micro-organisms such as Epstein–Barr and cytomegalovirus.

C. False. Biotin or digoxigenin can be used to give a colorimetric detection system.

D. False. ISH uses specific DNA probes.

E. True.

4.3 Autopsies:

A. Are being performed in increasing numbers on patients who die in British hospitals.

B. Are a useful audit of clinical diagnoses.

C. Provide useful epidemiological information.

D. Never provide material suitable for electron microscopy.

E. Are performed only for medicolegal purposes.

4.4 The following may be directly visualised using light microscopy:

A. Mitochondrial cristae.

B. Nuclei.

C. Oncogenes.

D. Fungi.

E. Bacteria.

(Answers overleaf)

4.3 **A.** **False.** In most British hospitals the rate of autopsies on patients who die in hospitals has fallen from about 60% to 25% during this century.

    B. **True.** Most studies show that up to 30% of clinical diagnoses are not confirmed at autopsy.

    C. **True.** The prevalence of many diseases can be assessed by careful autopsy studies.

    D. **False.** Although autolysis is a problem there is often sufficient preservation of subcellular organelles to make examination by electron microscopy possible if this is required.

    E. **False.** Autopsies may be performed for medicolegal purposes but may be performed with the consent of the deceased's relatives if a death certificate has been completed.

4.4 **A.** **False.** The internal structure of mitochondria requires the resolution which electron microscopy, but not light microscopy, can provide.

    B. **True.** Nuclei are easily seen using light microscopy, and details of the nucleus are very important in making histological diagnoses.

    C. **False.** Oncogenes are part of the nuclear DNA and cannot be directly visualised by any microscopic technique.

    D. **True.** Fungi can be seen by light microscopy, especially when special stains are used which react with fungal cell wall material.

    E. **True.** Bacteria are easily seen using light microscopy, the Gram stain being most widely used for this purpose.

5

Disorders of growth, differentiation and morphogenesis

5.1 Dysplasia is characterised by the following features:
- A. Evidence of decreased growth.
- B. Absence of cellular atypia.
- C. Loss of epithelial polarity.
- D. Increased number of mitotic figures.
- E. A low nuclear/cytoplasmic ratio.

5.2 The following conditions may cause muscular atrophy:
- A. Increased work-load.
- B. Denervation.
- C. Malnutrition.
- D. Ischaemia.
- E. Anabolic steroids.

5.3 The following genetic conditions result in proportional alteration of skeletal growth:
- A. Down's syndrome.
- B. Turner's syndrome.
- C. Achondroplasia.
- D. Pseudohypoparathyroidism.
- E. Beckwith–Weidemann syndrome.

(Answers overleaf)

5.1   **A.** **False.**   There is evidence of increased growth in dysplastic tissues as shown by increased tissue bulk and increased number of mitoses.
   B. **False.**   Cellular atypia is present in dysplastic tissues and is visualised as nuclear pleomorphism and hyperchromatism of nuclei.
   C. **True.**   Haphazard orientation of nuclei is a characteristic feature of dysplastic epithelium.
   D. **True.**   This is evidence of increased growth. The mitotic figures may be found in areas where they are normally absent, e.g. above the basal layer in dysplastic squamous epithelium.
   E. **False.**   The size of the nucleus in dysplastic cells is usually increased in relation to the cytoplasm.

5.2   **A.** **False.**   Increased work-load produces muscular hypertrophy.
   B. **True.**   This atrophy may be seen in conditions such as poliomyelitis.
   C. **True.**   Malnutrition, particularly protein deficiency, can produce muscular atrophy.
   D. **True.**   An example of this is Volkmann's ischaemic contracture of the forearm muscles.
   E. **False.**   Anabolic steroids produce an increase in muscle mass.

5.3   **A.** **True.**   In trisomy 21 there is proportional reduction in skeletal growth resulting in decreased adult stature.
   B. **True.**   The X0 genotype results in proportionally decreased skeletal growth.
   C. **False.**   Achondroplasia results in disproportionate shortening of the limb bones.
   D. **True.**   This rare X-linked dominant condition is characterised by insensitivity to parathyroid hormone and results in proportional decrease in skeletal growth.
   E. **True.**   There is proportional increased skeletal growth in this syndrome which is due to duplication of the short arm of chromosome 11.

5.4   Metaplastic change to a squamous epithelium may occur in the following circumstances:

   A.   Bronchi in cigarette smokers.
   B.   Appendix in appendicitis.
   C.   Prostate around areas of infarction.
   D.   Bladder in chronic cystitis.
   E.   Upper oesophagus in oesophagitis.

5.5   Hypertrophy of smooth muscle occurs in the following situations:

   A.   The uterus in pregnancy.
   B.   Urinary bladder with outflow obstruction.
   C.   Quadriceps muscle in a bodybuilder.
   D.   Breast lobule in pregnancy.
   E.   Colon proximal to a stenosing tumour.

5.6   The following factors are likely to produce a decrease in infant birthweight:

   A.   Maternal alcohol abuse.
   B.   Maternal tobacco abuse (20 cigarettes or more a day).
   C.   Maternal habitation at altitudes above 10 000 feet.
   D.   Maternal diabetes mellitus.
   E.   Maternal drug abuse.

(Answers overleaf)

5.4 **A.** **True.**   The ciliated columnar epithelium of the bronchi often undergoes metaplasia to squamous epithelium in cigarette smokers.

B. **False.**   The glandular epithelium of the appendix shows no propensity to undergo squamous metaplasia.

C. **True.**   It is important to recognise this as metaplasia and not invasive squamous carcinoma.

D. **True.**   The transitional epithelium of the bladder often changes to metaplastic squamous epithelium in conditions of chronic irritation.

E. **False.**   Since the upper oesophagus is lined by squamous epithelium it cannot undergo metaplasia to squamous epithelium.

5.5 **A.** **True.**   There is enormous hypertrophy of uterine smooth muscle during pregnancy. There is also a degree of hyperplasia.

B. **True.**   Outflow obstruction, usually in males due to benign nodular hyperplasia of the prostate, causes hypertrophy of bladder smooth muscle which is apparent as trabeculation of the bladder wall.

C. **False.**   Quadriceps is striated muscle.

D. **False.**   There are some myoepithelial cells in breast lobules but these undergo hyperplasia, rather than hypertrophy, during pregnancy.

E. **True.**   The smooth muscle in the colon will hypertrophy in response to the increased work-load of pushing the luminal contents through the stenosis.

5.6 **A.** **True.**   Maternal alcohol abuse retards fetal growth. Associated abnormalities include microcephaly, hypotonia, atrial septal defects and facial dysmorphology.

B. **True.**   Consumption of 20 cigarettes a day through pregnancy results in an average reduction in birthweight of 7%. Cigarette smoking probably reduces uterine blood flow.

C. **True.**   This effect of altitude may be due to decreased availability of intra-uterine oxygen.

D. **False.**   The average birthweight of infants born to mothers with diabetes mellitus is increased above the population norm.

E. **True.**   It is not clear whether this is a specific effect of the drugs or related to associated socioeconomic deprivation.

5.7   Male breast hypertrophy (gynaecomastia):
   A.   Is associated with hepatic cirrhosis.
   B.   Is due to hyperplasia of breast lobules.
   C.   Is associated with the treatment of prostatic carcinoma.
   D.   Is always bilateral.
   E.   May be caused by adrenal tumours.

5.8   Hyperplasia of the thyroid gland:
   A.   Occurs in Sheehan's syndrome.
   B.   Occurs in Graves' disease.
   C.   Is caused by increased levels of ACTH.
   D.   Occurs in thyroid dyshormonogenesis.
   E.   May be caused by a pituitary tumour.

5.9   Psoriasis:
   A.   Is a condition which is characterised by atrophy of the skin.
   B.   Shows elongation of the rete ridges on histological examination.
   C.   Affects about 2% of the population of Britain.
   D.   Is characterised by an increased rate of turnover of epidermal cells.
   E.   Is an infective disease.

(Answers overleaf)

5.7 **A. True.** Oestrogen levels are increased in hepatic cirrhosis and may induce gynaecomastia.
   B. False. The enlargement of the breasts in gynaecomastia is due to the increased amount of oedematous stromal tissue. Lobules do not occur in the male breast, only ductal structures are present.
   C. True. Oestrogens are sometimes used to treat metastatic prostatic carcinoma and these may induce gynaecomastia.
   D. False. Male breast hypertrophy may be unilateral.
   E. True. Some adrenal tumours secrete oestrogens and so can induce gynaecomastia.

5.8 **A. False.** In Sheehan's syndrome there is panhypopituitarism because the pituitary has infarcted. The reduced or absent production of thyroid stimulating hormone (TSH) results in thyroid atrophy.
   B. True. An auto-antibody is produced in Graves' disease which stimulates the TSH receptors of the thyroid leading to hyperplasia.
   C. False. ACTH (adrenocorticotrophic hormone) acts on the adrenal cortex; it has no effect on the thyroid.
   D. True. Defective production of thyroid hormones leads to a compensatory increase in TSH levels which cause thyroid hyperplasia.
   E. True. A TSH-producing pituitary tumour would cause thyroid hyperplasia, but such a tumour is very rare.

5.9 **A. False.** Psoriasis is characterised by hyperplasia of the skin.
   B. True. This is one of the characteristic histological features.
   C. True.
   D. True. The turnover of epithelial cells is at least twice as fast as that of normal skin.
   E. False. There is no known infective agent which causes psoriasis. The cause of psoriasis is unknown; some theories suggest that chalones (growth inhibitor substances) are not produced when the epidermis has attained its usual thickness.

5.10 Apoptosis:
- **A.** Involves the death of large contiguous areas of cells.
- **B.** Is caused by non-lysosomal endogenous endonuclease.
- **C.** Is a pathological event.
- **D.** May be seen in histological sections.
- **E.** Leaves a permanent clump of cellular debris.

5.11 Patau's syndrome:
- **A.** Affects 1 in 1000 births.
- **B.** Features prominent epicanthic folds.
- **C.** Features polydactyly.
- **D.** Features microphthalmia.
- **E.** Is caused by trisomy 13.

(Answers overleaf)

5.10   **A.   False.**   Apoptosis is the death of individual cells rather than of large adjacent groups of cells.

   B.   True.   This enzyme breaks down nuclear DNA into smaller fragments.

   C.   False.   Apoptosis is a physiological event which balances the production of new cells to produce a stable cellular population.

   D.   True.   Cells which have undergone apoptosis are seen as rounded membrane-bound bodies.

   E.   False.   These bodies are eventually phagocytosed and digested by adjacent cells so that they are not permanent.

5.11   **A.   False.**   Patau's syndrome occurs in 1 in 6000 births.

   B.   False.   This is a feature of trisomy 21 (Down's syndrome).

   C.   True.

   D.   True.

   E.   True.

6

Responses to cellular injury

6.1 **The following circumstances will inhibit repair of damaged tissue:**
- **A.** Scurvy.
- **B.** Hypothyroidism.
- **C.** Infection.
- **D.** Immobilisation.
- **E.** Ultraviolet light.

6.2 **The following tissues are likely to regenerate following damage:**
- **A.** Cerebral cortex.
- **B.** Myocardium.
- **C.** Bone.
- **D.** Liver.
- **E.** Spinal cord.

6.3 **Fibrinoid necrosis:**
- **A.** Occurs in arteriolar walls in malignant hypertension.
- **B.** Appears blue on haematoxylin and eosin staining.
- **C.** Is usually due to clostridial infection.
- **D.** Is caused by enzymatic lysis of adipose tissue.
- **E.** Is the characteristic appearance seen in tuberculosis.

(Answers overleaf)

6.1 **A.** **True.** Vitamin C is required for the synthesis of collagen.
  B. **True.** Healing is generally slowed in myxoedematous patients.
  C. **True.** Infection can be a potent inhibitor of healing.
  D. **False.** Immobilisation is beneficial in the healing of fractured bones and soft tissue injuries.
  E. **False.** It has been reported that ultraviolet light promotes healing of lesions such as skin wounds. It may do this by inhibiting infection.

6.2 **A.** **False.** After early life, neurones do not have the ability to replicate — so regeneration cannot occur.
  B. **False.** Myocytes cannot replicate, so regeneration is not possible. Damaged areas of myocardium are replaced by fibrous scar tissue.
  C. **True.** Bone has excellent properties of regeneration. Remodelling of fracture callus can produce complete restoration of a fractured bone.
  D. **True.** Liver cells are capable of regeneration. If damage to the liver continues whilst replication occurs, there may not be a complete return to original architecture, and if the damage is severe then cirrhosis may occur.
  E. **False.** Gliosis is the only reaction that the spinal cord can make to injury.

6.3 **A.** **True.** Fibrinoid necrosis, often seen in renal biopsies, is the histological hallmark of malignant hypertension.
  B. **False.** It appears as a bright pink (eosinophilic) colour on haematoxylin and eosin staining.
  C. **False.** Gas gangrene is usually caused by clostridial infection. No infectious agents are involved in the pathogenesis of fibrinoid necrosis.
  D. **False.** Enzymatic lysis of (or direct trauma to) adipose tissue results in fat necrosis with many foamy macrophages.
  E. **False.** The necrosis seen in tuberculosis is typically caseous.

6.4   **Granulation tissue:**
  A. Contains fibroblasts.
  B. Always contains granulomas.
  C. Often occurs after acute short-lived injury to the liver.
  D. Contains thin-walled capillaries.
  E. Actively contracts.

6.5   **The following factors will delay healing of a bony fracture:**
  A. Stabilisation.
  B. Infection.
  C. Misalignment.
  D. Interposed soft tissue.
  E. Paget's disease of bone.

6.6   **The acute effects of high-dose radiation exposure include:**
  A. Diarrhoea.
  B. Anaemia.
  C. Leukaemia.
  D. Endarteritis obliterans.
  E. Skin desquamation.

(Answers overleaf)

6.4   **A.** **True.**   These are important cells in the process of repair.
   B. **False.**   Granulation tissue derives its name from the granular appearance of the base of a skin ulcer. Granulomas are not an integral part of granulation tissue but may be present if there is foreign material or an infectious agent which elicits a granulomatous response.
   C. **False.**   Liver cells are capable of rapid regeneration, so healing by repair is an uncommon event in the liver unless the injury is persistent or repetitive.
   D. **True.**   These capillaries produce the granular appearance of the tissue.
   E. **True.**   Some of the fibroblasts differentiate into myofibroblasts, so active contraction of the granulation tissue is possible.

6.5   **A.** **False.**   Stabilisation of a fracture promotes healing because it prevents excessive callus formation.
   B. **True.**   Infection, such as may be acquired through the skin wound of a compound fracture, delays the healing of a fracture.
   C. **True.**   Although a small degree of malalignment will not affect fracture healing, any gross error in alignment will delay bony union.
   D. **True.**   Fractures can heal only when the two bony surfaces are opposed. Intervening soft tissue will prevent fracture healing.
   E. **True.**   Any pre-existing bone disease, such as Paget's disease or metastatic carcinoma, will delay healing of a fracture.

6.6   **A.** **True.**   The surface lining of the small intestine is renewed every 24–48 hours, so radiation damage will result in insufficient replacement of these cells, reduction in the absorptive surface area and consequent diarrhoea.
   B. **True.**   Depression of bone marrow activity by radiation can lead to an anaemia.
   C. **False.**   Leukaemia is a long-term effect of radiation damage. The mean delay for the development of leukaemia after the atomic explosions in Nagasaki and Hiroshima was 12.5 years.
   D. **False.**   This is a long-term effect of irradiation; it often accompanies tissue atrophy.
   E. **True.**   There may also be reddening of the skin (erythroderma) due to vasodilatation.

6.7   In cell death by apoptosis:

   A. Cell membrane integrity is lost.
   B. Death of contiguous cell groups occurs.
   C. An inflammatory response is usual.
   D. There is energy-dependent fragmentation of DNA by endogenous endonucleases.
   E. Lysosomes leak lytic enzymes.

(Answers overleaf)

6.7   **A.** **False.**   The integrity of the cell membrane is maintained during apoptosis, it is lost in cell death due to necrosis.

B. **False.**   Apoptosis results in death of single cells, groups of cells die in necrosis.

C. **False.**   There is usually no inflammatory response to apoptosis, which again contrasts with necrosis in which an inflammatory response is usual.

D. **True.**

E. **False.**   Lysosomes remain intact during apoptosis.

7

Disorders of metabolism and homeostasis

7.1 Amyloidosis:

A. Of AL type may complicate rheumatoid arthritis.
B. Occurs in about 15% of subjects with multiple myeloma.
C. May be diagnosed by rectal biopsy.
D. Of AA type may complicate chronic osteomyelitis.
E. If fatal, usually causes death by hepatic failure.

7.2 Phenylketonuria:

A. May be detected using the Guthrie test.
B. Is due to a deficiency of phenylalanine hydroxylase.
C. Is characterised by hyperpigmentation of the skin.
D. Occurs in 1 in 1000 infants in Britain.
E. Is characterised by mental retardation.

7.3 Dystrophic calcification:

A. May occur in the absence of any derangement of calcium metabolism.
B. May result in the formation of psammoma bodies.
C. Is associated with hyperparathyroidism.
D. Is associated with the ingestion of large amounts of milk.
E. May lead to heterotopic bone formation.

7.1 **A.** **False.** Amyloidosis may complicate rheumatoid arthritis, but it is the AA, rather than AL, type.

 B. **True.** The AL type of amyloidosis is a common complication of myelomatosis.

 C. **True.** The rectum is a relatively accessible site from which a biopsy can be taken; a rectal biopsy shows positive staining for amyloid in about 80% of cases of amyloidosis. The biopsy should include submucosa and muscle for the maximum chance of detecting amyloid.

 D. **True.** Chronic osteomyelitis was a common cause of amyloidosis; antibiotic therapy has reduced its incidence.

 E. **False.** Renal failure is the usual mode of dying if amyloidosis is fatal. Even when the liver contains much amyloid protein its function is relatively unimpaired.

7.2 **A.** **True.** The Guthrie test is a screening test performed on all neonates using blood obtained from a heel prick.

 B. **True.** This is the specific enzyme deficiency.

 C. **False.** Hypopigmentation of the skin is the characteristic feature.

 D. **False.** Phenylketonuria occurs at a rate of about 1 in 10 000 infants.

 E. **True.** If a subject with phenylketonuria receives a normal diet in infancy and childhood then mental retardation occurs due to damage by toxic metabolites of phenylalanine.

7.3 **A.** **True.** Dystrophic calcification is the deposition of calcium in damaged tissue; it usually occurs in individuals with normal calcium metabolism.

 B. **True.** Psammoma bodies are spherical laminated deposits of calcium. They are also found in tumours such as papillary carcinoma of the thyroid and meningiomas.

 C. **False.** Hyperparathyroidism may produce metastatic calcification.

 D. **False.** This may lead to the milk–alkali syndrome, with subsequent metastatic calcification.

 E. **True.** Dystrophic calcification of long standing may mature into heterotopic bone.

7.4 Homocystinuria:
- **A.** Is inherited in an autosomal dominant pattern.
- **B.** Is characterised by mental retardation.
- **C.** Produces a habitus of similar form to Marfan's syndrome.
- **D.** Is due to a deficiency of homogentisic acid oxidase.
- **E.** Produces hepatomegaly.

7.5 Gout:
- **A.** Is more common in females than males.
- **B.** Is more frequent in those with low, rather than high, socioeconomic status.
- **C.** May produce subcutaneous tophi.
- **D.** Is characterised by hypouricaemia.
- **E.** Causes an acute arthritis.

7.6 Amyloid protein:
- **A.** Gives an apple-green birefringence when stained with Congo red and examined by polarised light.
- **B.** Has an alpha-helical chain structure.
- **C.** Is deposited intracellularly.
- **D.** Stains with Lugol's iodine.
- **E.** Is a soluble protein.

7.7 Hyponatraemia:
- **A.** Is a feature of Cushing's syndrome.
- **B.** Is a feature of Addison's disease.
- **C.** Commonly occurs in renal failure.
- **D.** Causes an increase in blood volume.
- **E.** May result from excessive diuretic therapy.

(Answers overleaf)

7.4 **A. False.** Homocystinuria is inherited, like most other inherited disorders of metabolism, in an autosomal recessive pattern.
  B. True. Fits may also be a feature.
  C. True. Homocystine accumulates and interferes with the cross-linking of collagen and elastic fibres.
  D. False. Cystathione synthetase is the deficient enzyme in homocystinuria. Homogentisic acid oxidase is deficient in alkaptonuria.
  E. False. Hepatomegaly is a feature of the storage diseases, such as the mucopolysaccharidoses, but is not a feature of homocystinuria.

7.5 **A. False.** Gout is more common in men than women.
  B. False. Gout is more common in those with higher socioeconomic status.
  C. True. These tophi are deposits of urate crystals.
  D. False. Gout is characterised by *hyper*uricaemia.
  E. True. This arthritis characteristically affects the first metatarsophalangeal joint.

7.6 **A. True.** This is the most widely-used means of identification, and the apple-green birefringence is highly specific for amyloid.
  B. False. Amyloid has a beta-pleated sheet structure.
  C. False. It is deposited extracellularly.
  D. True. Amyloid stains dark brown with Lugol's iodine; this is a useful macroscopic indication of amyloid deposition.
  E. False. Amyloid protein is insoluble and is resistant to digestion by proteases, so once deposited it is likely to persist.

7.7 **A. False.** The increased production of glucocorticoids in Cushing's syndrome causes *hyper*natraemia.
  B. True. Hyponatraemia is a characteristic biochemical feature of Addison's disease. A low serum cortisol would confirm the diagnosis.
  C. False. Hypernatraemia (and hyperkalaemia) are among the usual biochemical features of renal failure.
  D. False. Hyponatraemia causes a decrease in blood volume.
  E. True. Another complication of certain types of diuretic therapy is hypokalaemia.

7.8   Thiamine (B₁) deficiency:

A. Is associated with alcoholism.

B. May produce confusion and amnesia with confabulation.

C. Causes a peripheral neuropathy.

D. May cause cardiac failure.

E. Causes subacute combined degeneration of the spinal cord.

7.9   Hypercalcaemia:

A. Often occurs after surgical removal of the parathyroid glands.

B. May cause metastatic calcification of tissues.

C. Often causes polyuria.

D. May be caused by a deficiency of vitamin D.

E. May cause vomiting.

7.10   Wilson's disease:

A. Is due to a deficiency of body copper.

B. Is inherited in an autosomal recessive pattern.

C. May be diagnosed by the presence of Kayser–Fleischer rings.

D. May cause hepatic cirrhosis.

E. May be treated with D-penicillamine.

7.11   Cystic fibrosis:

A. Is inherited in an autosomal recessive pattern.

B. Is due to mutations in a transmembrane conductance regulator.

C. Is associated with chronic pancreatitis.

D. Is associated with recurrent bronchopulmonary infections.

E. Has no effect on male fertility.

(Answers overleaf)

7.8 **A. True.** Alcoholism is the most common predisposing factor in Britain; a deficient diet associated with the excessive consumption of alcohol is the most likely cause.

B. True. This group of symptoms is known collectively as Korsakoff's psychosis.

C. True. This is a characteristic feature.

D. True. If cardiac failure is a feature then the disease is sometimes called 'wet beri-beri'.

E. False. Vitamin B_{12} deficiency leads to subacute combined degeneration of the spinal cord.

7.9 **A. False.** Surgical removal of the parathyroid glands causes a deficiency of parathyroid hormone and subsequent *hypo*calcaemia.

B. True. This is a feature of long-standing hypercalcaemia.

C. True. This is a characteristic feature of hypercalcaemia.

D. False. Hypercalcaemia may be caused by hypervitaminosis D.

E. True. Fits may also occur.

7.10 **A. False.** Wilson's disease is due to an accumulation of copper in the body.

B. True.

C. True. These rings are present around the corneal limbus.

D. True. A chronic hepatitis is frequently present and may lead to cirrhosis.

E. True. D-penicillamine is a chelating agent which will remove the accumulated copper but it cannot reverse the hepatic and cerebral damage which may have occurred.

7.11 **A. True.**

B. True.

C. True. This may present in adult life.

D. True. This is due to the viscid secretions retained in the bronchi.

E. False. Males with cystic fibrosis usually have reduced fertility.

8

Ischaemia, infarction and shock

8.1 **The macroscopic appearances of postmortem blood clot include:**

    A. Lines of Zahn.
    B. Shiny surface.
    C. Separation of red blood cells and plasma producing a 'chicken fat' appearance.
    D. Adherence to vessel walls.
    E. Friability.

8.2 **These factors predispose to the formation of venous thromboses:**

    A. Immobility.
    B. The oral contraceptive pill.
    C. Heparin therapy.
    D. Polycythaemia rubra vera.
    E. Thrombocytopenia.

(Answers overleaf)

8.1   **A.** **False.**   The lines of Zahn are seen in antemortem thrombus, rather than postmortem blood clot. The pale lines are platelet aggregates, whilst the intervening dark lines are composed of red blood cells enmeshed in fibrin.

B. **True.**   Postmortem blood clot often has a shiny surface, in contrast to the dull surface of blood clot formed before death.

C. **True.**   Red blood cells often gravitate to the bottom of postmortem blood clot, leaving the separated plasma to give a 'chicken fat' appearance.

D. **False.**   Adherence to the vessel wall is a characteristic of antemortem thrombosis; postmortem blood clot usually peels easily from the vessel in which it lies.

E. **True.**   Postmortem blood clot is usually more friable than that formed during life.

8.2   **A.** **True.**   Immobility from any cause (post-operative, chronic illness, prolonged air travel) predisposes to venous thrombosis.

B. **True.**   There is some increase in the incidence of venous thrombosis amongst women taking the oral contraceptive pill. This effect is thought to be related to the amount of oestrogen in the pill, so the risk with modern low-dose oestrogen pills is very small.

C. **False.**   Heparin therapy reduces the incidence of venous thrombosis.

D. **True.**   Polycythaemia rubra vera increases the coagulability of the blood and so is associated with an increased incidence of venous thrombosis.

E. **False.**   Thrombocytopenia may produce a bleeding diathesis.

8.3   **Pulmonary embolism:**

  A.   Often produces strain on the left side of the heart.
  B.   Is a common intra-operative complication.
  C.   Always produces pulmonary infarction.
  D.   Is usually associated with a thrombosis in the deep veins of the legs or the pelvic veins.
  E.   May cause sudden death.

8.4   **An embolus in the arterial system may originate from:**

  A.   A myxoma in the left atrium.
  B.   An atheromatous plaque.
  C.   A venous thrombosis.
  D.   A prosthetic pulmonary valve.
  E.   Air entering a venous cannula.

8.5   **The following organs have two different systems of blood supply:**

  A.   Spleen.
  B.   Liver.
  C.   Kidney.
  D.   Lung.
  E.   Prostate.

(Answers overleaf)

8.3 **A.** **False.** It is the right side of the heart which has an increased work-load in pulmonary embolism.

      B. **False.** Pulmonary embolism rarely occurs intra-operatively but it is a significant post-operative complication.

      C. **False.** The lungs have a dual blood supply from the pulmonary and bronchial arteries, so that infarction is not an invariable accompaniment of pulmonary embolism.

      D. **True.** A thrombosis in the leg or pelvic veins is the commonest source of a pulmonary embolus.

      E. **True.** A significant proportion of almost instantaneous deaths are due to pulmonary embolism. Many occur in immobile individuals with other illness, but sometimes sudden death from pulmonary embolism occurs in individuals without predisposing factors.

8.4 **A.** **True.** The first manifestation of such a tumour may be embolic phenomena.

      B. **True.** Atheromatous plaques in the aorta may ulcerate and produce emboli which may produce infarcts in distal organs.

      C. **True.** This is an uncommon occurrence since the embolus can gain access to the arterial system only through a patent foramen ovale or atrial septal defect.

      D. **False.** There is no pathway for an embolus from a valve in the pulmonary position to get into the arterial system; emboli would be filtered out in the lungs.

      E. **True.** This can occur only in the circumstances mentioned in C, above.

8.5 **A.** **False.** The spleen has a single arterial supply, so occlusion of this supply often leads to splenic infarction.

      B. **True.** The liver has a dual supply from the portal vein and hepatic artery.

      C. **False.** The kidney is another organ with a single supply and is therefore susceptible to infarction.

      D. **True.** The lung is supplied by the pulmonary and bronchial arteries.

      E. **False.** The prostate is a fairly common site of infarction, particularly when enlarged through benign prostatic hyperplasia.

8.6   **The following agents promote thrombolysis:**

  A. Warfarin.
  B. Fibrinogen.
  C. Streptokinase.
  D. Plasmin.
  E. α_1-Antitrypsin.

8.7   **The fat embolism syndrome:**

  A. Is associated with severe skeletal injuries.
  B. Usually manifests itself within 12 hours of injury.
  C. Is fatal in over 80% of cases.
  D. Is associated with thrombocythaemia.
  E. May be definitively diagnosed in routine paraffin-embedded sections.

8.8   **Amniotic fluid embolism:**

  A. Is commoner in primigravidae.
  B. Occurs in about 1 in 5000 deliveries.
  C. Often causes disseminated intravascular coagulation.
  D. Is fatal in 85–95% of cases.
  E. Is associated with prolonged labour.

8.9   **The following vascular lesions may cause ischaemia:**

  A. Hypoviscosity.
  B. Vasculitis.
  C. Atheroma.
  D. Spasm.
  E. Compression.

(Answers overleaf)

8.6 **A. False.** Warfarin prevents the formation of thrombus by decreasing the amount of vitamin K-dependent clotting factors, but it does not possess fibrinolytic activity.
  B. False. Fibrinogen is a precursor of fibrin, which is involved in the formation of thrombus.
  C. True. Streptokinase is used as a therapeutic fibrinolytic agent.
  D. True. Plasmin acts on fibrin to produce soluble degradation products.
  E. False. α_1-Antitrypsin inhibits the action of plasmin.

8.7 **A. True.** Fat emboli may be demonstrated in 90% of cases of severe skeletal injury but the syndrome of fat embolism is less common.
  B. False. The symptoms usually appear 24–72 hours after the initiating injury.
  C. False. The fat embolism syndrome has a fatal outcome in about 10% of cases.
  D. False. Thrombocytopenia often occurs.
  E. False. Frozen sections are required to demonstrate fat emboli because fat dissolves in the solvents used in paraffin-embedding techniques.

8.8 **A. False.** Amniotic fluid embolism is commoner in multiparous women.
  B. False. It occurs in 1 in 50 000 to 80 000 deliveries.
  C. True. Extensive fibrin thrombi are found in small vessels.
  D. True. If amniotic fluid embolism produces clinical manifestations then it is frequently fatal.
  E. False. Amniotic fluid embolism is associated with abrupt, precipitous labour.

8.9 **A. False.** *Hyper*viscosity of the blood, as may occur in hypergammaglobulinaemia, can cause impaired flow and predisposes to thrombosis.
  B. True. Inflammation in a vessel wall narrows its lumen and may be complicated by superimposed thrombosis.
  C. True. Atheroma only occurs in arteries, by itself it narrows vessel lumina, which may lead to ischaemia, and it may be complicated by thrombosis and embolism.
  D. True. Contraction of the smooth muscle in the media of a vessel may lead to ischaemia.
  E. True. Veins are especially subject to this because their walls are thinner than those of arteries.

8.10 The following may occur as a consequence of shock:

- **A.** Acute tubular necrosis.
- **B.** Acute pancreatitis.
- **C.** Irreversible neuronal injury.
- **D.** Cerebral haemorrhage.
- **E.** Subendocardial myocardial infarction.

(Answers overleaf)

8.10   **A.   True.**   This may lead to acute renal failure but the tubules can regenerate — if shock is reversed renal function will usually return within a couple of weeks.

B.   True.

C.   True.

D.   False.   Cerebral infarction may occur, especially in the 'watershed' areas between the adjacent territories of cerebral arteries.

E.   True.

9

Immunology and immunopathology

9.1   Immunoglobulins of M class (IgM):
 A. Cross the placenta.
 B. Are characteristically produced in a secondary immune response.
 C. Are usually found as a dimeric form linked by a J chain.
 D. Can activate complement.
 E. Are usually found bound to the surface of mast cells.

9.2   T-lymphocytes:
 A. Produce antibodies.
 B. Mature in the thymus.
 C. Are identified by the presence of surface immunoglobulin.
 D. Produce lymphokines.
 E. May be subdivided into helper and suppressor/cytotoxic subtypes.

9.3   The classical pathway of complement activation:
 A. Is activated by lipopolysaccharide cell wall constituents.
 B. Starts with the activation of the C1 component.
 C. Is activated by IgA immune complexes.
 D. Is activated by IgG which has bound to its specific antigen.
 E. Is activated by IgM which has bound to its specific antigen.

9.1 **A. False.** IgM cannot cross the placenta, so if IgM antibodies directed against infectious organisms are found in the fetal blood then they are an indicator of intra-uterine infection.

B. False. IgM antibodies are characteristic of a primary immune response; IgG antibodies predominate in a secondary immune response.

C. False. IgM is usually found in a pentameric form. IgA is usually found as a dimer linked by a J chain.

D. True. IgM is an effective activator of complement when it has bound to its specific antigen.

E. False. IgE is the class of antibody which is usually found bound to the surface of mast cells.

9.2 **A. False.** B-lymphocytes, which have differentiated into plasma cells, produce antibodies.

B. True. Hence the designation T-lymphocytes. B-lymphocytes derive their prefix from the bursa of Fabricius, which is where they mature in chickens (humans do not have a bursa of Fabricius).

C. False. B-lymphocytes have surface immunoglobulin. T-lymphocytes were originally identified by their ability to bind red blood cells in a rosette formation; the method currently used involves monoclonal antibodies directed against cell surface antigens.

D. True. Lymphokines are chemical messengers which regulate the proliferation of other lymphocytes.

E. True.

9.3 **A. False.** The alternative pathway of complement activation is initiated by these endotoxins.

B. True. The cascade sequence then progresses through C4, 2, 3, 5, 6, 7, 8 and 9.

C. False. These complexes activate complement by the alternative pathway.

D. True.

E. True.

9.4   **Immediate (type I) hypersensitivity:**

A.   May be prevented by administration of disodium chromoglycate.

B.   Is caused by antigen reacting with IgM antibodies.

C.   May cause death.

D.   Has a positive association with the Wiskott–Aldrich syndrome.

E.   Is characterised by the Arthus reaction.

9.5   **Interleukin-1 (IL-1):**

A.   Stimulates hepatocytes to synthesise acute phase proteins.

B.   Stimulates laying down of new bone.

C.   Inhibits the release of neutrophils from the bone marrow.

D.   Causes prostaglandin-induced proteolysis in muscle.

E.   Activates fibroblasts.

9.6   **The human major histocompatibility complex:**

A.   Is situated on chromosome 4.

B.   Is also known as the HLA complex.

C.   Codes for blood group antigens.

D.   Is involved in transplant rejection.

E.   Codes for two classes of antigens which are expressed on all nucleated cells.

(Answers overleaf)

9.4 **A.** **True.** Disodium chromoglycate stabilises the membrane of mast cells thus preventing their degranulation and release of chemical mediators such as histamine.

B. **False.** Type I hypersensitivity is caused by antigen binding to IgE on the surface of mast cells and basophil leukocytes.

C. **True.** Acute systemic anaphylaxis, caused by antigen entering the blood and reacting with basophil leukocytes, can lead to death from circulatory collapse and bronchial constriction.

D. **True.** Wiskott–Aldrich syndrome is a rare inherited defect of T-cell function and is strongly associated with atopy. This indicates that regulation of the immune response by T-cells is important in prevention of hypersensitivity reactions.

E. **False.** The Arthus reaction is a feature of type III hypersensitivity reactions.

9.5 **A.** **True.**

B. **False.** IL-1 stimulates osteoclasts to reabsorb bone.

C. **False.** IL-1 stimulates the release of neutrophils from the bone marrow.

D. **True.**

E. **True.**

9.6 **A.** **False.** The major histocompatibility complex in humans is located on chromosome 6.

B. **True.** The major histocompatibility antigens are most easily detected on leukocytes, so it is also known as the human leukocyte antigen (HLA) system.

C. **False.**

D. **True.** If the MHC antigens are completely matched (such as transplants between monozygotic twins) then rejection does not occur.

E. **False.** There are two classes of HLA antigens (classes I and II) but only class I is expressed on all nucleated cells.

9.7   Immune complex (type III) hypersensitivity:
- **A.** Is mediated by specifically-sensitised T-lymphocytes.
- **B.** Causes myasthenia gravis.
- **C.** May occur in systemic lupus erythematosus.
- **D.** May cause a glomerulonephritis.
- **E.** May cause allergic asthma.

9.8   Hyperacute rejection:
- **A.** Occurs 2–4 days after transplantation.
- **B.** Is a cell-mediated response.
- **C.** May be minimised by blood group matching.
- **D.** Never occurs in autografts.
- **E.** May be reversed by cyclosporin A.

9.9   HLA matching is not required in these types of organ transplants:
- **A.** Cornea.
- **B.** Bone.
- **C.** Kidney.
- **D.** Bone marrow.
- **E.** Liver.

(Answers overleaf)

9.7 **A. False.** Type III hypersensitivity is mediated by antibodies. Type IV hypersensitivity is mediated by specifically-sensitised T-lymphocytes.

  B. False. Myasthenia gravis is caused by antibodies which bind to, and block, the acetylcholine receptors on skeletal muscle. No complexes of antigen and antibody are involved, so this represents a type II, rather than a type III, hypersensitivity response.

  C. True. Immune complexes between nuclear antigens and IgG antibodies may be formed in SLE in large amounts and result in a type III hypersensitivity reaction.

  D. True. Immune complexes may deposit in the glomerular basement membrane and cause a glomerulonephritis.

  E. False. Allergic asthma is a type I hypersensitivity reaction. Extrinsic allergic alveolitis ('farmers' lung' etc.) is a respiratory disease caused by a type III hypersensitivity reaction.

9.8 **A. False.** It occurs within minutes of transplantation.

  B. False. It is due to preformed cytotoxic antibodies.

  C. True. The cytotoxic antibodies are usually directed against blood group antigens.

  D. True. The blood groups and HLA antigens of autografts will be identical.

  E. False. Cyclosporin can suppress chronic rejection but cannot reverse hyperacute rejection.

9.9 **A. True.** The cornea is an immunologically 'privileged' site, so host lymphocytes do not gain access to the graft, and HLA matching is not required.

  B. True. Bone grafts are used as a scaffold for the ingrowth of host tissue, so its viability is not important.

  C. False. HLA matching produces better graft survival in kidney transplantation.

  D. False. HLA matching is required to prevent graft-versus-host disease.

  E. True.

9.10 Graft-versus-host disease:

- **A.** May cause cholestatic liver disease.
- **B.** Often causes a characteristic dermatitis.
- **C.** May be reduced by selective destruction of graft T-lymphocytes.
- **D.** May produce malabsorption.
- **E.** Is a common complication of renal transplantation.

9.11 Acquired immune deficiency syndrome (AIDS):

- **A.** May be transmitted vertically during childbirth or breast feeding.
- **B.** Is associated with *Pneumocystis carinii* pneumonia.
- **C.** Is associated with Kaposi's sarcoma.
- **D.** Affected about 10 million people worldwide in 1999.
- **E.** Is caused by Herpes simplex virus.

(Answers overleaf)

9.10 **A.** **True.** Bile ducts express class II HLA antigens, and so may be destroyed during graft-versus-host disease.
B. **True.**
C. **True.** A more effective way of reducing the incidence of graft-versus-host disease is by careful HLA matching at as many loci as possible.
D. **True.** Enterocytes are destroyed in graft-versus-host disease, producing malabsorption and diarrhoea.
E. **False.** Graft-versus-host disease occurs after bone marrow transplantation. The host immune system readily kills any graft lymphocytes remaining in a kidney after transplantation.

9.11 **A.** **True.**
B. **True.**
C. **True.**
D. **False.** About 33 million people were living with HIV infection in 1999.
E. **False.** It is caused by the human immunodeficiency virus (HIV).

10

Inflammation

10.1 Neutrophil polymorphs:
- **A.** Have bilobed nuclei.
- **B.** Are the predominant cell type in chronic inflammation.
- **C.** May fuse to form multinucleated giant cells.
- **D.** Have phagocytic abilities.
- **E.** Have numerous eosinophilic granules in their cytoplasm.

10.2 The following organisms characteristically induce a granulomatous inflammatory response:
- **A.** *Mycobacterium tuberculosis.*
- **B.** *Staphylococcus aureus.*
- **C.** *Treponema pallidum.*
- **D.** *Mycobacterium leprae.*
- **E.** *Streptococcus pneumoniae.*

10.3 The following are oxygen-independent killing mechanisms present in neutrophils:
- **A.** Lysozyme.
- **B.** Lactoferrin.
- **C.** Myeloperoxidase.
- **D.** Cationic proteins.
- **E.** Hydrogen peroxide.

(Answers overleaf)

10.1 **A. False.** Neutrophil polymorphs have multilobed rather than bilobed nuclei.

   B. False. Neutrophils are present in large numbers in acute inflammation; in chronic inflammation other cells predominate.

   C. False. Macrophages (synonyms: monocytes, histiocytes) have this ability.

   D. True. The phagocytic ability of neutrophil polymorphs plays a vital role in defence against bacterial infection.

   E. False. Neutrophils are included in the group of granulocytic cells but their granules are not eosinophilic.

10.2 **A. True.** Tuberculosis is the archetypal granulomatous disease.

   B. False. *Staph. aureus* causes an acute suppurative response without granuloma formation.

   C. True. Granulomas are a characteristic feature of syphilis.

   D. True. Granulomas are most prevalent in the tuberculoid form of leprosy.

   E. False. *Strep. pneumoniae*, the causative organism of many lobar pneumonias, causes an acute inflammatory response of which granulomas are not a feature.

10.3 **A. True.** Lysozyme (muramidase) damages the bacterial cell wall.

   B. True. Lactoferrin chelates iron so that none is available for bacterial growth.

   C. False. Myeloperoxidase is part of the oxygen-dependent pathway for killing micro-organisms in neutrophils.

   D. True.

   E. False. Hydrogen peroxide is the substrate upon which myeloperoxidase acts to produce peroxide anions, hydroxyl radicals and singlet oxygen.

10.4 **A neutrophil leukocytosis is characteristic of infections with these agents:**

  A. Epstein–Barr virus.
  B. *Brucella abortus.*
  C. *Streptococcus pneumoniae.*
  D. *Bordetella pertussis.*
  E. *Neisseria meningitidis.*

10.5 **Macrophages:**

  A. Have phagocytic, but not pinocytic, abilities.
  B. Are derived from blood monocytes.
  C. Have a shorter life-span than neutrophils.
  D. Contain neutral proteases.
  E. Produce interleukin-1.

10.6 **The following substances are found in the specific granules in the cytoplasm of human neutrophils:**

  A. Myeloperoxidase.
  B. Cationic proteins.
  C. Lactoferrin.
  D. Elastase.
  E. Lysozyme.

10.7 **Bradykinin:**

  A. Is formed from a precursor by the action of kallikrein.
  B. Directly initiates fibrinolysis.
  C. Causes decreased vascular permeability.
  D. Is stored in mast cells.
  E. Is also known as factor XII.

(Answers overleaf)

10.4 **A.** **False.** A lymphocytosis (increased number of lymphocytes in the blood) is the usual blood picture in infectious mononucleosis.

B. **False.** Undulant fever (brucellosis) usually produces a lymphocytosis.

C. **True.** Increased numbers of neutrophils are usually found in the blood of subjects infected with this organism.

D. **False.** Whooping cough usually produces a lymphocytosis.

E. **True.** Meningococcal meningitis is usually accompanied by a neutrophil leukocytosis.

10.5 **A.** **False.** Macrophages are able to ingest material by both phagocytic and pinocytic pathways.

B. **True.** Labelling experiments have confirmed that macrophages are derived from blood monocytes.

C. **False.** Macrophages have a much longer life-span than neutrophils.

D. **True.** These neutral proteases include plasminogen activator, collagenase and elastase.

E. **True.** Interleukin-1 is thought to have many activities including lymphocyte activation and pyrexia production.

10.6 **A.** **False.** Myeloperoxidase is found in the larger azurophilic intracytoplasmic granules.

B. **False.** Cationic proteins are also found in the larger azurophilic granules. These cationic proteins include those which increase vascular permeability and attract monocytes.

C. **True.** Lactoferrin is an iron-binding protein which may play a role in defence against some bacterial infections.

D. **False.** Elastase is found in the larger azurophilic granules. Other similar enzymes found in these granules include collagenases and cathepsin.

E. **True.** Lysozyme has antibacterial properties.

10.7 **A.** **True.** Kallikrein acts on kininogen to form bradykinin.

B. **False.** Plasmin is the main fibrinolytic factor.

C. **False.** Bradykinin is a potent increaser of vascular permeability.

D. **False.** Bradykinin is a plasma protein; it is not stored in cells.

E. **False.** Factor XII is Hageman factor.

10.8 **These are examples of primary chronic inflammation:**
 A. Unresolving lobar pneumonia.
 B. Sarcoidosis.
 C. Appendiceal abscess mass.
 D. Tuberculosis.
 E. Leprosy.

10.9 **Langhans' giant cells:**
 A. Are the antigen-presenting cells present in skin.
 B. Have a central ring of nuclei with clear peripheral cytoplasm.
 C. Are characteristically seen in tuberculosis.
 D. Have nuclei scattered randomly through their cytoplasm.
 E. Are derived from macrophages.

10.10 **The following substances are recognised chemical mediators of inflammation:**
 A. Histamine.
 B. Prostaglandin E_1.
 C. Dopamine.
 D. Amiodarone.
 E. Kallidin.

(Answers overleaf)

10.8 **A.** **False.**   Although chronic inflammatory cells may be present in a lobar pneumonia which has been present for some time, there will have been an initial phase of acute inflammation, so it is best regarded as secondary chronic inflammation.

   B. **True.**   There is no known preceding acute inflammatory phase in sarcoidosis.

   C. **False.**   This will have had an initial phase of acute inflammation.

   D. **True.**   Tuberculosis begins as a chronic inflammatory response.

   E. **True.**   Another mycobacterial infection which produces chronic, rather than acute, inflammation.

10.9 **A.** **False.**   The antigen-presenting cells present in skin are Langerhans' cells.

   B. **False.**   These are the histological features of Touton giant cells which are seen in areas of fat necrosis and lipomas.

   C. **True.**   They may be seen in other forms of granulomatous inflammation.

   D. **False.**   Foreign-body giant cells have this pattern of nuclear distribution.

   E. **True.**   They are thought to arise by fusion of macrophages when several of these cells attempt to engulf simultaneously an exogenous particle.

10.10 **A.** **True.**   Histamine produces vasodilatation and increased vascular permeability.

   B. **True.**   Prostaglandin E_1 (PGE_1) also produces vasodilatation and increased vascular permeability.

   C. **False.**   Dopamine is a neurotransmitter substance. It does not act as a chemical mediator of inflammation.

   D. **False.**   Amiodarone is an anti-arrhythmic drug.

   E. **True.**   Kallidin and bradykinin are kinins formed from plasma precursors. In inflammation they cause vasodilatation and increased vascular permeability.

11

Carcinogenesis and neoplasia

11.1 **The following mechanisms may cause a qualitative change in the expression of a gene:**

A. Gene amplification.
B. Chromosomal rearrangement.
C. Enhancer insertion.
D. Point mutation.
E. Promoter insertion.

11.2 **Gatekeeper genes:**

A. Maintain the integrity of the genome by repairing DNA damage.
B. Inhibit the proliferation, or promote the death, of cells with damaged DNA.
C. Are exemplified by the *p53* gene.
D. Are mutated in familial retinoblastoma.
E. Are exemplified by the *BRCA1* gene.

11.3 **An increased frequency of tumours caused by Ionising radiation has been demonstrated in the following groups:**

A. Aniline dye workers.
B. Luminous watch-dial painters.
C. Residents of Nagasaki in 1945.
D. Plutonium miners.
E. Caucasians resident in Queensland, Australia.

(Answers overleaf)

11.1 **A.** **False.** Gene amplification results in an increase in gene expression, a quantitative change.

B. **True.** Chromosomal rearrangement may result in a qualitative change in a gene, e.g. translocation involving chromosomes 9 and 22 in chronic myeloid leukaemia (Philadelphia chromosome) results in a fusion of c-*abl* and *bcr* genes to produce a protein with tyrosine kinase activity.

C. **False.** An enhancer sequence, inserted downstream from a gene, results in increased expression of a gene without a qualitative change in its product.

D. **True.** A point mutation may lead to a qualitative change in a gene and gene product. Examples in human tumours are the range of mutations that have been found in the Harvey *ras* gene.

E. **False.** A promoter sequence, inserted upstream from a gene, gives a similar effect to enhancer insertion.

11.2 **A.** **False.** It is caretaker genes that perform this function.

B. **True.**

C. **True.** This gene codes for a transcription factor and is mutated in about 50% of human cancers.

D. **True.** The *Rb1* gene was one of the first gatekeeper genes to be identified.

E. **False.** *BRCA1* is an example of a caretaker gene.

11.3 **A.** **False.** There is an increased incidence of bladder cancer in workers in the aniline dye industry but this is due to chemical carcinogens and not to ionising radiation.

B. **True.** About 10% of workers who painted watch dials with luminous radium-containing paint developed bone sarcomas. They ingested the radium as they pointed their brushes using their mouths.

C. **True.** There has been a high incidence of leukaemia in survivors of the atomic bomb blast in Nagasaki.

D. **True.** There is an increased frequency of lung carcinoma amongst plutonium miners.

E. **False.** There is a high incidence of skin tumours amongst the Caucasian residents of Queensland but this is due to ultraviolet light rather than ionising radiation.

11.4 **The Epstein–Barr virus (EBV) has a proven positive association with the following conditions:**

A. Carcinoma of the cervix.
B. Infectious mononucleosis.
C. Human T-cell lymphoma.
D. Burkitt's lymphoma.
E. Undifferentiated nasopharyngeal carcinoma.

11.5 **The following chemicals are strongly implicated as carcinogens for the tumours listed next to them:**

A. β-Naphthylamine — bladder cancer.
B. Vinyl chloride — hepatic angiosarcoma.
C. Aflatoxins — lung cancer.
D. Androgenic steroids — vaginal adenocarcinoma.
E. Cyclophosphamide — leukaemia.

11.6 **The following neoplasms have been shown to be associated with a consistent chromosomal defect:**

A. Meningiomas.
B. Burkitt's lymphoma.
C. Chronic myeloid leukaemia.
D. Retinoblastoma.
E. Wilms' tumour.

(Answers overleaf)

11.4 **A. False.** There is no described association between EBV and carcinoma of the cervix. The human papillomaviruses do have a strong association with this tumour.
B. True. EBV is the causative agent of infectious mononucleosis.
C. False. A T-cell lymphoma/leukaemia in the Caribbean and Japan has been shown to be associated with HTLV I.
D. True. Burkitt's lymphoma in malaria-ridden areas of Africa has a strong association with EBV.
E. True. Nasopharyngeal carcinoma has a positive association with EBV.

11.5 **A. True.** Benzidine and 4-aminobiphenyl are other chemical carcinogens implicated in the causation of bladder cancer.
B. True. Exposure to vinyl chloride monomer has a strong association with hepatic angiosarcoma.
C. False. Aflatoxins are implicated in the causation of some cases of hepatocellular carcinoma.
D. False. Prenatal exposure to diethylstilboestrol (an oestrogenic steroid) is associated with vaginal adenocarcinoma. Androgenic anabolic steroids are associated with liver tumours.
E. True. There is a small, but proven, risk of leukaemia in humans who have received cyclophosphamide therapy.

11.6 **A. True.** About 90% of meningiomas have some deletion from the long arm of chromosome 22. If the deletion is large the meningioma tends to be more aggressive.
B. True. A translocation between chromosomes 8 and 14 is common. This translocation puts the c-*myc* proto-oncogene next to busy immunoglobulin genes.
C. True. The Philadelphia chromosome (chromosome 22 with a deletion) is present in about 90% of cases of chronic myeloid leukaemia.
D. True. A deletion from chromosome 13 is often associated with retinoblastoma.
E. True. A deletion from chromosome 11 has been described in Wilms' tumour.

11.7 **Phaeochromocytoma has an increased incidence in the following inherited conditions:**

  A. Multiple endocrine neoplasia (MEN) syndromes.
  B. Familial polyposis coli.
  C. Von Hippel–Lindau syndrome.
  D. Familial retinoblastoma.
  E. Xeroderma pigmentosum.

11.8 **In cell culture, features which characterise transformed cells include:**

  A. Loss of contact inhibition of growth.
  B. Loss of density inhibition of growth.
  C. Production of plasminogen activator.
  D. Diploid chromosome content.
  E. Limited life-span of the culture.

11.9 **In England and Wales during the 1990s:**

  A. Lung carcinoma was the commonest malignant tumour in women.
  B. Gastric carcinoma had a higher incidence than colorectal carcinoma.
  C. Carcinoma of the oesophagus was less common than carcinoma of the bladder.
  D. Carcinoma of the ovary was a rare tumour in females.
  E. Pancreatic carcinoma was more common than prostatic carcinoma in males.

(Answers overleaf)

11.7 **A. True.**
  B. False. Colorectal carcinoma and other intestinal tumours have an increased incidence in familial polyposis coli.
  C. True. Other tumours which have an increased incidence in this condition are cerebellar haemangioblastoma and renal cell carcinoma.
  D. False.
  E. False. Skin cancers have an increased incidence in this condition.

11.8 **A. True.** Normal cells tend to stop growing when they are touching other cells.
  B. True. Untransformed cells form a monolayer in culture, transformed cells form multilayered heaps.
  C. True. Plasminogen activator may assist in tumour invasion.
  D. False. Transformed cells usually have an aneuploid chromosomal complement.
  E. False. Transformed cell cultures often continue growing indefinitely ('immortalisation') whereas untransformed cells have a finite life-span.

11.9 **A. False.** It is important to have some knowledge of the relative incidence of various tumours, and this knowledge is vital to those who plan the overall health care system in Britain. Carcinoma of the breast was the commonest malignant tumour in women in the 1990s with 27% of cases; lung carcinoma was ranked third but was rapidly closing on colorectal cancer for second place.
  B. False. Colorectal carcinoma was more common than gastric carcinoma in both men and women.
  C. True. This difference was more marked in men than in women. Bladder carcinoma was three times more common than oesophageal carcinoma in males.
  D. False. Carcinoma of the ovary was the fourth most common tumour in females, both in incidence and mortality.
  E. False. Prostatic carcinoma was the second most frequent carcinoma in males, with three times as many cases as pancreatic carcinoma, which ranked ninth.

11.10 Sarcomas:

A. Are more common than carcinomas.

B. Metastasise more commonly by lymphatic than haematogenous routes.

C. Have a long *in-situ* phase.

D. Have a peak incidence in those below 50 years of age.

E. Are derived from connective tissues.

11.11 The following malignant neoplasms rarely metastasise:

A. Bronchial carcinoma.

B. Breast carcinoma.

C. Astrocytomas.

D. Renal cell carcinoma.

E. Cutaneous basal cell carcinomas.

11.12 In the TNM staging system for tumours:

A. M1 indicates that distant metastases are present.

B. pNX indicates that the regional lymph nodes cannot be assessed histologically.

C. The T component indicates the extent of the primary tumour.

D. N2 denotes many nodal metastases.

E. In Hodgkin's disease the staging is synonymous with the Ann Arbor classification.

(Answers overleaf)

11.10 A. False. Carcinomas are much more common than sarcomas.
   B. False. The preferred route of metastasis is the blood; this contrasts with carcinomas, which usually metastasise by the lymphatics.
   C. False. No *in-situ* phase has been identified for sarcomas. In carcinomas there is often an *in-situ* phase.
   D. True.
   E. True.

11.11 A. False. It is estimated that about 50% of bronchial carcinomas have metastasised by the time of clinical presentation.
   B. False. Breast carcinoma metastasises very readily to sites such as lung, bone and brain.
   C. True. Astrocytomas, even the poorly-differentiated glioblastoma multiforme, rarely metastasise within the central nervous system and metastasise outside this area only if there is an artificial connection such as a ventriculoperitoneal shunt.
   D. False. Renal cell carcinomas characteristically invade the renal veins and extend into the inferior vena cava, so blood-borne metastases are common.
   E. True. Basal cell carcinomas (rodent ulcers) are locally invasive, but they metastasise very infrequently.

11.12 A. True. M0 indicates absence of distant metastases.
   B. True. All stages assessed by histological examination are prefixed by a 'p'.
   C. True.
   D. True. N0 indicates no nodal metastases, N1 one or a few nodal metastases, and N2 many nodal metastases.
   E. False. A TNM system has not been applied to Hodgkin's disease. The Ann Arbor classification is the standard system used in this disease.

11.13 Benign, rather than malignant, tumours are characterised by the following features:
  A. Increased numbers of mitotic figures.
  B. Microinvasion.
  C. Nuclear pleomorphism.
  D. Well-ordered maturation.
  E. Ability to metastasise.

11.14 The following tumours are benign:
  A. Lymphangioma.
  B. Liposarcoma.
  C. Wilms' tumour.
  D. Seminoma.
  E. Osteoma.

11.15 The following definitions are correct:
  A. An adenoma is a benign tumour of glandular epithelium.
  B. A carcinoma is a malignant epithelial tumour.
  C. Neoplasia means new growth.
  D. A leiomyoma is a benign tumour of striated muscle.
  E. A polyp is a neoplastic pedunculated mass attached to a surface.

11.16 The following cysts are neoplastic:
  A. Hydatid cysts.
  B. Cystadenomas.
  C. Branchial cysts.
  D. Cystic teratoma.
  E. Thyroglossal cysts.

(Answers overleaf)

11.13 A. False. Benign tumours generally contain fewer mitotic figures than do malignant tumours.
B. False. Any breach of the basement membrane is strong evidence that a tumour is malignant rather than benign.
C. False. Nuclear pleomorphism (variation in nuclear size) is a more prominent feature of malignant, as opposed to benign, tumours.
D. True. Malignant tumours usually show a disorder of maturation.
E. False. Ability to metastasise is the key feature of malignant tumours.

11.14 A. True. A lymphangioma is a benign tumour derived from lymph vessels.
B. False. A liposarcoma is a malignant tumour with differentiation towards fat cells.
C. False. Wilms' tumour (nephroblastoma) is a malignant tumour derived from the renal anlage.
D. False. Seminomas are malignant tumours which are thought to be derived from germ cells.
E. True. An osteoma is a benign bone tumour.

11.15 A. True. A papilloma is a benign tumour arising from squamous, basal or transitional type epithelium.
B. True. A carcinoma is a malignant epithelial tumour.
C. True.
D. False. A leiomyoma is a benign tumour of *smooth* muscle. A rhabdomyoma is a benign tumour of striated muscle.
E. False. A polyp is a pedunculated mass attached to a surface but it is not necessarily neoplastic.

11.16 A. False. Hydatid cysts are caused by the parasite *Taenia echinococcus*.
B. True. These are benign cystic neoplasms of glandular epithelium; the most commonly recognised site is the ovary.
C. False. These are congenital cysts due to embryological defects.
D. True. These germ cell tumours occur mainly in the gonads.
E. False. These are congenital cysts, again arising from embryological defects.

11.17 The following tumours and eponymous names are correctly matched:

A. Burkitt's lymphoma — a T-cell lymphoma common in Europe.

B. Kaposi's sarcoma — a vascular neoplasm associated with AIDS.

C. Wilms' tumour — an embryonal tumour of the kidney.

D. Grawitz tumour — adrenocortical carcinoma.

E. Ewing's sarcoma — a malignant tumour of bone of uncertain histogenesis.

11.18 The following tumours are APUDomas:

A. Pancreatic carcinoma.

B. Medullary carcinoma of the thyroid.

C. Phaeochromocytoma.

D. Appendiceal carcinoid tumour.

E. Gastrinoma.

(Answers overleaf)

11.17 A. False. The reaction of doctors and students to eponymous medical terms is mixed. Some like the idea of medical history being represented in the names of diseases and find them easy to remember; others (perhaps with more rigorously scientific minds) insist that a name should describe the disease. Burkitt's lymphoma is obviously a neoplasm of lymphoid origin but it has B-cell differentiation and is most common in areas of endemic malaria in Africa.

B. True. This neoplasm was rare until the AIDS epidemic but was found in an endemic form in Africa.

C. True.

D. False. Grawitz tumour is another name for renal cell carcinoma. This tumour has many synonyms, including clear cell carcinoma of the kidney and, confusingly, hypernephroma (because of its microscopic resemblance to adrenal tissue).

E. True.

11.18 A. False. Pancreatic carcinoma arises from the epithelial cells in the exocrine part of the pancreas. Insulinomas are pancreatic APUDomas but arise from cells in the islets of Langerhans.

B. True. This tumour was described before the concept of APUDomas was formulated; calcitoninoma would be a more logical name.

C. True. These tumours may produce paroxysmal hypertension.

D. True.

E. True. These tumours arise from gastrin-producing cells.

12

Ageing and death

12.1 **The following are valid criteria for the diagnosis of brainstem death:**
  A. Absence of corneal reflex.
  B. Argyll Robertson pupil sign.
  C. Gag reflex is present.
  D. No respiratory effort occurs when the patient is disconnected from a mechanical ventilator for 30 seconds.
  E. The vestibulo-ocular reflexes are absent.

12.2 **These pathologies often cause death to occur very suddenly (within a few minutes at longest):**
  A. Ruptured myocardial infarct.
  B. Cerebral infarct.
  C. Ruptured aortic aneurysm.
  D. Subarachnoid haemorrhage.
  E. Meningococcal meningitis.

12.3 **Telomeres:**
  A. Are situated in the centromeric regions of chromosomes.
  B. Lengthen with each cell division.
  C. Are non-coding tandemly repetitive sequences of DNA.
  D. Are replicated by the enzyme telomerase.
  E. Are prematurely shortened in progeria.

(Answers overleaf)

12.1 **A.** **True.**

B. **False.** The Argyll Robertson pupil sign occurs in living subjects and is a sign of neurosyphilis. The pupils are fixed in diameter and do not react to light when there is brainstem death.

C. **True.**

D. **False.** There is no set period from disconnection from the ventilator; ventilation should cease for long enough for the measured arterial carbon dioxide level to rise above the threshold required to stimulate respiration.

E. **True.**

12.2 **A.** **True.** The pericardial sac becomes distended with blood producing cardiac tamponade.

B. **False.** If cerebral infarction causes death it usually does so after several hours or a day or two because the major reason for death is raised intracranial pressure caused by oedema around the area of infarction.

C. **True.** The entire blood volume is rapidly lost into the retroperitoneum, peritoneum or thoracic cavity when an aortic aneurysm ruptures.

D. **True.**

E. **False.** There are a few hours between the onset of infection and death (if it is fatal) in meningococcal meningitis so there is a good chance of recovery if appropriate antibiotics are given in this period.

12.3 **A.** **False.** Telomeres are situated at the tips of each chromosome.

B. **False.** Telomeres shorten with each cell division in most cells and stay the same length in germ cells (which possess telomerase).

C. **True.**

D. **True.**

E. **True.**

13

Cardiovascular system

13.1 Infective endocarditis:

A. In intravenous drug abusers commonly affects the tricuspid valve.
B. May produce a microcytic hypochromic anaemia.
C. If caused by streptococci has a mortality rate of over 50%.
D. Usually affects more than one heart valve.
E. Often produces a shift to the right in granulocytes.

13.2 Atrial septal defect (ASD):

A. Is the commonest congenital cardiac anomaly.
B. Is associated with Down's syndrome.
C. Usually causes death before puberty if untreated.
D. May lead to pulmonary hypertension.
E. Occurs more frequently in males than females.

13.3 The following are major risk factors for the development of atherosclerosis:

A. Cigarette smoking.
B. Hypocholesterolaemia.
C. Hypertension.
D. Diabetes insipidus.
E. Male sex.

(Answers overleaf)

13.1 **A.** **True.**   The tricuspid valve is affected in over half the intravenous drug abusers who develop infective endocarditis.

B. **True.**   This occurs secondary to intravascular haemolysis.

C. **False.**   Streptococcal endocarditis can be eradicated in over 90% of cases using appropriate antibiotic therapy.

D. **False.**   A single valve, predominantly the aortic or mitral, is affected in 80–90% of cases.

E. **False.**   A left shift, towards more immature forms, is the usual blood picture in infective endocarditis.

13.2 **A.** **False.**   ASDs account for about 10% of congenital cardiac anomalies. Ventricular septal defects are more frequent, with 25% of the total.

B. **True.**   Most congenital cardiac anomalies have an increased incidence in Down's syndrome.

C. **False.**   Survival to middle age is usual, even without surgical correction.

D. **True.**   Pulmonary hypertension may occur because of increased pulmonary blood flow due to the left-to-right shunt.

E. **False.**   ASD is more common in females than males.

13.3 **A.** **True.**   Studies have shown that smoking 20 cigarettes a day increases the risk of atherosclerosis sufficient to cause three times the normal incidence of ischaemic heart disease.

B. **False.**   *Hyper*cholesterolaemia is a major risk factor. Population studies show that increased plasma cholesterol has a direct relationship with increased incidence of atherosclerosis.

C. **True.**   Increase in both diastolic and systolic blood pressure has been shown to be associated with an increased incidence of atherosclerosis.

D. **False.**   Diabetes *mellitus* is a major risk factor for atherosclerosis.

E. **True.**   Pre-menopausal females rarely suffer from advanced atherosclerosis.

13.4 **There is an increased incidence of deep venous thrombosis in the following states:**
 A. Pregnancy.
 B. Carcinoma of the pancreas.
 C. Oral contraceptive administration.
 D. Advanced age.
 E. Congestive cardiac failure.

13.5 **In malignant hypertension:**
 A. Renin levels are decreased.
 B. There may be a microangiopathic haemolytic anaemia.
 C. Arterioles often show fibrinoid necrosis.
 D. Papilloedema is rare.
 E. With treatment, the 5-year survival rate is about 10%.

13.6 **Aschoff bodies:**
 A. Contain fibroblasts.
 B. May contain Anitschokow cells.
 C. Are found exclusively in the heart.
 D. Are always associated with active rheumatic fever.
 E. May contain Askanazy cells.

(Answers overleaf)

13.4 A. True.   The incidence is highest in the third trimester. The predisposition is due to hypercoagulability and inhibition of fibrinolysis.
B. True.   This association was first recorded by Trousseau. The thromboses often appear and regress in different areas.
C. True.   The strongest association appears to be with the oestrogen content of the pill.
D. True.   This is probably due to the decreased mobility which tends to accompany increased age.
E. True.   Congestive cardiac failure is associated with venous congestion and decreased mobility.

13.5 A. False.   Renin levels are markedly increased due to renal ischaemia.
B. True.   Mechanical trauma to red blood cells often leads to intravascular haemolysis.
C. True.   This fibrinoid necrosis is the histological hallmark of malignant hypertension (compare this with the hyaline arteriolosclerosis of benign hypertension).
D. False.   Papilloedema (with retinal exudates and haemorrhages) is a common ophthalmoscopic finding in malignant hypertension.
E. False.   With good treatment, the 5-year survival rate is about 50%. Without treatment most subjects die within a few months.

13.6 A. True.   Fibroblasts appear in Aschoff bodies during the proliferative phase of their development.
B. True.   These cells have a peculiar pattern of nuclear chromatin which gives them the alternative name of 'caterpillar cells'.
C. False.   Aschoff bodies may also be found in synovium, tendons and other connective tissues.
D. False.   Aschoff bodies may be found in subjects with no signs of active rheumatic fever. Either the bodies persist for a long time after periods of activity or latent disease may produce no clinical signs or symptoms.
E. False.   Askanazy cells are found in Hashimoto's thyroiditis.

13.7 Thrombo-angiitis obliterans (Buerger's disease):
  A. Often causes thrombosis in the tibial arteries.
  B. Is associated with cigarette smoking.
  C. Usually affects those older than 60 years.
  D. Leads to fibrous encasement of neurovascular bundles.
  E. Has an increased incidence in individuals with HLA haplotypes A9 and B5.

13.8 Aortic aneurysms of atherosclerotic origin:
  A. Are more common in males than females.
  B. Are more common in the aortic arch than the descending aorta.
  C. Rarely contain mural thrombus.
  D. Often rupture when greater than 60 mm in diameter.
  E. May occlude the renal arteries.

13.9 The following features are described as part of Fallot's tetralogy:
  A. Atrial septal defect.
  B. Patent ductus arteriosus.
  C. Right ventricular hypertrophy.
  D. Ventricular septal defect.
  E. Displacement of the aorta to the right.

(Answers overleaf)

13.7 **A.** **True.** The radial arteries are the other common site of thrombosis.

B. **True.** Thrombo-angiitis obliterans rarely occurs in non-smokers.

C. **False.** The peak incidence occurs between the ages of 25 and 50 years.

D. **True.** Extension of the inflammation from arteries into surrounding veins and nerves leads to fibrous encasement of neurovascular bundles which is a characteristic histological feature.

E. **True.** Genetic factors are also implicated by the higher incidence in India, Japan and Israel.

13.8 **A.** **True.** Men are affected five times more commonly than women.

B. **False.** Atherosclerotic aneurysms are commonest in the abdominal aorta. Syphilitic aneurysms more frequently affect the aortic arch.

C. **False.** Mural thrombus is commonly present and may completely fill a saccular aneurysm.

D. **True.** Approximately 80% of subjects with aneurysms of greater than 60 mm diameter die of rupture of their aneurysm within 10 years if left untreated.

E. **True.** The iliac and mesenteric arteries are also vulnerable.

13.9 **A.** **False.**

B. **False.**

C. **True.** The right ventricular hypertrophy is secondary to stenosis of the pulmonary outflow tract.

D. **True.** There will be a right-to-left shunt through this defect, producing cyanosis.

E. **True.**

13.10 The following conditions may lead to secondary hypertension:
  A. Hypothyroidism.
  B. Hyperaldosteronism.
  C. Addison's disease.
  D. Phaeochromocytoma.
  E. Renal artery stenosis.

13.11 Polyarteritis nodosa:
  A. Is associated with chronic carriage of hepatitis B virus.
  B. Is a necrotising vasculitis.
  C. Commonly affects the kidneys.
  D. Affects females more commonly than males.
  E. Affects predominantly large arteries.

13.12 Fatty streaks in the aorta:
  A. Contain lipid which is predominantly extracellular.
  B. Often appear in the first year of life.
  C. Contain a proliferation of smooth muscle cells.
  D. Are rare in Third World populations.
  E. Are usually greater than 10 mm in diameter.

(Answers overleaf)

13.10 A. False. Hypertension may be a feature of *hyper*thyroidism.
  B. True. Hyperaldosteronism (Conn's syndrome) may cause secondary hypertension by increased retention of sodium and water.
  C. False. *Hypo*tension is a feature of Addison's disease due to deficiencies of glucocorticoids and mineralocorticoids.
  D. True. Phaeochromocytoma, a tumour of the adrenal medulla, may produce secondary hypertension which often has a paroxysmal nature.
  E. True. A marked degree of renal artery stenosis will produce renal ischaemia with increased renin secretion leading to secondary hypertension.

13.11 A. True. There is an increased incidence of hepatitis B surface antigen in the serum of subjects with polyarteritis nodosa.
  B. True. There is fibrinoid necrosis of all layers of the vessel wall.
  C. True. Autopsy studies have shown renal involvement in 80% of fatal cases.
  D. False. Males are more commonly affected than females in a ratio of 2:1.
  E. False. Medium- and small-size muscular arteries are the principal sites of the disease.

13.12 A. False. The lipid is predominantly intracellular within the cytoplasm of foamy macrophages.
  B. True. Fatty streaks often occur before the age of one year, most commonly in the ascending aorta and dorsal aspect of the descending aorta.
  C. False. A proliferation of smooth muscle cells occurs in established atherosclerotic plaques; it is not a feature of fatty streaks.
  D. False. Fatty streaks have a world-wide distribution, even in populations where established atherosclerosis is uncommon.
  E. False. Fatty streaks are usually a few millimetres wide and less than 10 mm in diameter.

13.13 Patent ductus arteriosus:
A. Is associated with intra-uterine rubella infection.
B. Occurs more commonly in males than females.
C. May cause death from infective endocarditis.
D. Is usually the only anomaly present.
E. May produce a heart murmur with a 'machinery-like' quality.

13.14 The following factors may acutely exacerbate ischaemic heart disease:
A. Platelet aggregation.
B. Thrombosis.
C. Arterial spasm.
D. Haemorrhage into an atherosclerotic plaque.
E. Hypotension.

13.15 The following features are likely to be present when a myocardial infarct of 24 hours' duration is examined by light microscopy:
A. Distortion of mitochondrial cristae.
B. Oedema.
C. A heavy infiltrate of neutrophils in the interstitium.
D. Total coagulative necrosis with loss of nuclei.
E. Haemorrhage.

(Answers overleaf)

13.13 A. True. PDA is also associated with prematurity and infantile respiratory distress syndrome.
B. False. PDA occurs more frequently in females than in males.
C. True. Death may also occur from right-sided heart failure in middle age.
D. False. Although PDA may be the only anomaly it is usually seen in association with other anomalies, such as transposition of the great vessels, where the shunt may improve the haemodynamic situation.
E. True. A continuous systolic/diastolic murmur with a harsh quality is characteristic of a PDA.

13.14 A. True. Platelet aggregation over an atherosclerotic plaque may further narrow a coronary artery and cause more ischaemia in the dependent myocardium.
B. True. Thrombosis over an atherosclerotic plaque may completely occlude a coronary artery and cause infarction of the distal myocardium.
C. True. Spasm may produce transient occlusion of coronary arteries and cause Prinzmetal's angina.
D. True. Capillary vessels within an atherosclerotic plaque may rupture, and the consequent haemorrhage may increase the degree of narrowing produced by the plaque.
E. True. Systemic hypotension superimposed on pre-existing atherosclerosis may lead to myocardial infarction.

13.15 A. False. This is an ultrastructural feature that would be detectable only by electron microscopy.
B. True. Interstitial and cellular oedema may be present.
C. True. Neutrophils are present in infarcts of 24 hours' duration.
D. False. Total coagulative necrosis, with loss of nuclei, is not apparent until about 72 hours.
E. True. Interstitial haemorrhage may be present at 24 hours.

13.16 These conditions may occur as complications of infective endocarditis:

A. Libman–Sacks endocarditis.
B. Diffuse proliferative glomerulonephritis.
C. Erosion of the chordae tendineae.
D. Intracerebral infarction.
E. Marantic vegetations.

13.17 Familial hypercholesterolaemia:

A. Is found in about 10% of the population.
B. In the homozygous form may produce death from myocardial infarction before the age of 20 years.
C. Is caused by deficient high-density lipoprotein (HDL) receptors.
D. In the heterozygous form is not associated with an increased incidence of atherosclerosis.
E. Is associated with raised triglyceride levels.

13.18 Dissecting aortic aneurysms:

A. Have an increased incidence in subjects with Marfan's syndrome.
B. Have a peak incidence in the third decade of life.
C. Usually originate from intimal tears around atheromatous plaques.
D. Have an untreated mortality of about 90%.
E. May lead to a 'double-barrelled' aorta.

(Answers overleaf)

13.16 A. False. This sterile endocarditis occurs in systemic lupus erythematosus.

B. True. This glomerulonephritis is thought to arise as an immune complex disease.

C. True. This can lead to prolapse of the mitral valve leaflets and acute cardiac embarrassment.

D. True. Cerebral infarction may occur as a result of embolisation of vegetations into the cerebral circulation.

E. False. Marantic vegetations are sterile vegetations which occur in cachectic states such as advanced malignancy.

13.17 A. False. It is found in about 1 in 500 of the population.

B. True. Homozygous individuals have a very high incidence of ischaemic heart disease secondary to coronary artery atherosclerosis.

C. False. It is lack of normal low-density lipoprotein (LDL) receptors that causes this condition.

D. False. Plasma cholesterol levels of heterozygotes are two to three times greater than normal, and there is an increased incidence of ischaemic heart disease in middle age.

E. False. Triglyceride levels are normal.

13.18 A. True. 'Cystic medial necrosis' of the aorta (mucinous degeneration and elastic fibre fragmentation) occurs in Marfan's syndrome and predisposes to dissecting aneurysms.

B. False. Most cases occur in elderly individuals.

C. False. Although the intimal tear may occur around an atheromatous plaque it most commonly occurs in disease-free areas of aortic intima.

D. True. A mortality of 90% within a week occurs in untreated cases. Treatment is usually directed at reducing systemic blood pressure to prevent further propagation of the dissection.

E. True. If the dissection re-enters the aorta then a 'double-barrelled' aorta may occur.

13.19 Cranial (giant-cell) arteritis:
- **A.** Has a positive association with polymyalgia rheumatica.
- **B.** May cause blindness.
- **C.** Is usually diagnosed by serological testing.
- **D.** Can be treated by administration of glucocorticoids.
- **E.** Only affects arteries in the head and neck.

13.20 These are complications of myocardial infarction:
- **A.** Dressler's syndrome.
- **B.** Ventricular arrhythmias.
- **C.** Pericarditis.
- **D.** Mitral incompetence.
- **E.** Ventricular aneurysm.

13.21 Mitral incompetence:
- **A.** May be caused by rheumatic fever.
- **B.** Produces an ejection systolic murmur.
- **C.** Has a positive association with ankylosing spondylitis.
- **D.** Produces a collapsing pulse.
- **E.** May be caused by mucoid degeneration of the mitral valve cusps.

(Answers overleaf)

13.19 **A.** **True.** Polymyalgia rheumatica accompanies cranial arteritis in about 50% of cases.

B. **True.** If the disease affects the ophthalmic or posterior ciliary arteries then blindness may result.

C. **False.** The disease is diagnosed clinically or by histological examination of the superior temporal artery.

D. **True.** The disease usually responds well to steroid therapy.

E. **False.** Any artery in the body may be affected but those in the head and neck are most commonly affected.

13.20 **A.** **True.** This syndrome (of chest pain, fever and effusions) is thought to be due to antibodies formed against previously 'unseen' cardiac antigens.

B. **True.** These may cause sudden death in the first few hours following infarction and are one of the reasons for the establishment of coronary care units with continuous electrocardiographic monitoring.

C. **True.** This occurs with transmural infarction.

D. **True.** This may occur with rupture of infarcted papillary muscles.

E. **True.** Infarcted muscle may be replaced by fibrous tissue which is stretched to form an aneurysm.

13.21 **A.** **True.**

B. **False.** The murmur is pansystolic. An ejection systolic murmur occurs in aortic stenosis.

C. **False.** Aortic incompetence is associated with the aortic root dilation that may occur in ankylosing spondylitis.

D. **False.** A collapsing pulse occurs in aortic incompetence.

E. **True.** This mucoid degeneration can lead to mitral valve prolapse and subsequent mitral valve incompetence.

13.22 The following agents may cause a myocarditis:
   A. Group B coxsackieviruses.
   B. Poliovirus.
   C. *Trypanosoma cruzi.*
   D. Ionising radiation.
   E. Adriamycin.

13.23 Pulseless (Takayasu's) disease:
   A. Usually affects cranial arteries.
   B. May cause hypertension.
   C. Is characterised by a necrotising arteritis.
   D. Affects males more commonly than females.
   E. Has a better prognosis than cranial (giant-cell) arteritis.

13.24 Atrial myxomas:
   A. Arise in the right atrium more commonly than in the left.
   B. Are the most frequent primary cardiac tumours.
   C. May cause ischaemia of the lower limbs.
   D. Are thought to represent organised thrombus.
   E. Are associated with signs of mitral valve disease.

(Answers overleaf)

13.22 A. True. Group A coxsackieviruses are also fairly common causes of myocarditis.
  B. True. The poliovirus causes myocarditis less commonly than the coxsackieviruses.
  C. True. This form of myocarditis is common in South America.
  D. True. Myocarditis may complicate therapeutic irradiation for thoracic malignancies.
  E. True. Other cytotoxic drugs, such as doxorubicin, can cause a myocarditis and this may have important implications for treatments such as high-dose chemotherapy followed by bone marrow transplantation.

13.23 A. False. Takayasu's disease affects the aorta and its proximal branches.
  B. True. Involvement of the renal arteries may cause hypertension, which may be difficult to control.
  C. True. The histological appearances are similar to those of cranial (giant-cell) arteritis.
  D. False. Young or middle-aged females are most commonly affected.
  E. False. The response to steroids is not usually as marked as with cranial (giant-cell) arteritis.

13.24 A. False. Three-quarters of atrial myxomas are situated in the left atrium.
  B. True. All other primary cardiac tumours are very rare; they include lipomas, rhabdomyomas, rhabdomyosarcomas and angiosarcomas.
  C. True. Material from left atrial myxomas can embolise and cause ischaemia in the lower limbs (so all embolectomy material should be submitted for histological examination).
  D. False. Intracardiac myxomas are thought to arise as tumours of undifferentiated connective tissue cells in the sub-endocardial layers of the heart wall.
  E. True. Signs and symptoms of mitral valve disease are present in about half the cases of atrial myxoma.

14

Respiratory tract

14.1 The following cells are found in the respiratory bronchioles:

A. Clara cells.
B. Chondrocytes.
C. Ciliated epithelial cells.
D. Type I pneumocytes.
E. Type II pneumocytes.

14.2 Subjects in these situations are more likely to have hyperplastic carotid bodies than is an ordinary person living at sea level:

A. Inhabitants of the Peruvian Andes.
B. People with Pickwickian syndrome.
C. People with acute allergic asthma.
D. People with kyphoscoliosis.
E. Olympic marathon runners.

14.3 The following respiratory function tests usually have reduced values in asthmatic subjects:

A. Peak expiratory flow rate (PEFR).
B. Vital capacity (VC).
C. Carbon monoxide transfer (TCO).
D. Forced expiratory ratio (FEV_1/VC).
E. Forced expiratory ratio in 1 second (FEV_1).

14.1 **A. True.** Clara cells secrete a proteinaceous fluid.
   B. False. There is no cartilage in bronchioles; it is present in the upper part of the respiratory tree in the trachea and bronchi.
   C. True. Ciliated epithelial cells line the bronchioles.
   D. False. Type I pneumocytes are found in the alveoli.
   E. False. Type II pneumocytes are found also in the alveoli where they secrete surfactant and are the stem cells for type I pneumocytes.

14.2 **A. True.** The high altitude of the Andes produces a decrease in arterial oxygenation and a secondary hyperplasia of the carotid bodies.
   B. True. The Pickwickian syndrome consists of gross obesity producing decreased chest movement and alveolar hypoventilation.
   C. False. Asthma is a reversible obstruction of the airways, so although there may be intermittent arterial hypoxaemia, this will not be sustained for long enough to produce hyperplasia of the carotid bodies.
   D. True. Severe kyphoscoliosis may produce chronic hypoventilation due to restriction of chest movement.
   E. False. Olympic marathon runners (along with cross-country skiers) have some of the highest recorded capacities for oxygen uptake, so arterial hypoxaemia will be very unlikely to occur.

14.3 **A. True.** This parameter is reduced in obstructive airways disease such as asthma.
   B. False. The vital capacity is usually normal in asthmatic subjects. It is reduced in restrictive respiratory disease such as pulmonary fibrosis.
   C. False. The carbon monoxide transfer is reduced in interstitial lung disease such as pulmonary fibrosis; it is usually normal in asthmatic subjects.
   D. True. The forced expiratory ratio is low in obstructive respiratory disease.
   E. True. This is often a more reliable measure of obstructive airways disease than is the peak expiratory flow rate.

14.4 **The following factors predispose to infections of the respiratory tract:**

  A. Coma.
  B. Immotile cilia syndromes.
  C. Congenital hypogammaglobulinaemia.
  D. Pulmonary oedema.
  E. Cystic fibrosis.

14.5 **Carcinoma of the larynx:**

  A. Is usually of adenocarcinomatous type.
  B. Is commoner in men than in women.
  C. Is associated with exposure to tobacco smoke.
  D. Has a treated 5-year survival rate of about 50%.
  E. May be complicated by lung infections.

14.6 **Malignant mesothelioma of the pleura:**

  A. In Europe, is related to asbestos exposure in about 20% of cases.
  B. Is associated with cigarette smoking.
  C. Has been decreasing in incidence in Britain during the 1980s.
  D. Often has a biphasic epithelial/sarcomatous pattern of differentiation on histological examination.
  E. Usually contains asbestos bodies.

(Answers overleaf)

14.4 **A.** **True.** Loss of the cough reflex during coma (or anaesthesia) can allow organisms entry to the lungs.
B. **True.** Impairment of cilia motility, such as occurs in Kartagener's syndrome, will predispose to respiratory infection.
C. **True.** Lack of antibodies in this condition reduces the efficiency of phagocytosis and of the killing of bacteria.
D. **True.** Flooding of the alveoli by oedema fluid increases the risk of respiratory infection.
E. **True.** The increased viscosity of mucous secretions in cystic fibrosis makes clearance of organisms from the respiratory tract more difficult.

14.5 **A.** **False.** 95% of laryngeal carcinomas show squamous cell differentiation.
B. **True.** It is seven times more frequent in males than in females.
C. **True.** Most cases of laryngeal carcinoma occur in smokers.
D. **True.** Presentation is probably earlier than comparable bronchial tumours, usually with symptoms of hoarseness, and so survival is much better when the condition is treated. The usual treatment is irradiation with or without laryngectomy.
E. **True.** Ulcerated tumours of the larynx are a potent source of infected debris in the distal airways.

14.6 **A.** **False.** In Europe about 90% of malignant pleural mesotheliomas are associated with asbestos exposure.
B. **False.** There is no conclusive evidence to implicate cigarette smoking in the causation of malignant mesothelioma, unlike the multiplicative effect of cigarette smoking to the risk of developing lung cancer in those exposed to asbestos.
C. **False.** The incidence of the tumour is expected to increase until the end of the century despite reductions in asbestos exposure. This is due to the long latent period between asbestos exposure and tumour formation (thought to be 20–50 years).
D. **True.** This is the characteristic histological pattern.
E. **False.** Asbestos bodies are rarely found within the malignant mesothelioma but are very commonly found in the underlying lung tissue.

14.7 Lobar pneumonia:

A. Affects females more commonly than males.
B. Is common in infancy and old age.
C. Is usually due to *Streptococcus pneumoniae.*
D. Passes through the stage of grey hepatisation before red hepatisation.
E. Is rarely associated with sputum production.

14.8 *Pneumocystis carinii* pneumonia:

A. Usually occurs in immunocompetent subjects.
B. Gives a histological picture of a foamy pink alveolar exudate.
C. May be diagnosed by cytological examination of bronchoalveolar lavage.
D. Is rarely life-threatening.
E. May be associated with other respiratory infections.

14.9 Adult respiratory distress syndrome (ARDS):

A. May be caused by ingestion of paraquat.
B. May be caused by high concentrations of inspired oxygen.
C. Can lead to an interstitial fibrosis.
D. Produces hyaline membranes which line the alveoli.
E. May lead to proliferation of type I pneumocytes.

(Answers overleaf)

14.7 **A.** **False.**   Males are affected more commonly than females.
       B. **False.**   Lobar pneumonia occurs most commonly in adults between the ages of 30 and 50 years.
       C. **True.**   About 90% of cases of lobar pneumonia are due to *Streptococcus pneumoniae.*
       D. **False.**   The stage of red hepatisation (when the alveoli are filled with red blood cells and neutrophils) precedes that of grey hepatisation (when there is abundant intra-alveolar fibrin).
       E. **False.**   Sputum is often plentiful and may have a rusty colour due to flecks of blood.

14.8 **A.** **False.**   *Pneumocystis* pneumonia usually occurs in the immunocompromised, especially those with AIDS.
       B. **True.**   This is the characteristic histological appearance.
       C. **True.**   Silver impregnation stains make identification of the organism relatively easy in cytological preparations.
       D. **False.**   *Pneumocystis* pneumonia is a common terminal event in AIDS.
       E. **True.**   Other opportunistic infections, such as those caused by cytomegalovirus or *Aspergillus*, may be present.

14.9 **A.** **True.**   Paraquat is a potent lung toxin. Other drugs which, in overdosage, may cause ARDS include barbiturates and diamorphine.
       B. **True.**   Oxygen toxicity, due to formation of free oxygen radicals, may occur with inspired oxygen concentrations of over 70%.
       C. **True.**   Although ARDS may resolve to leave a relatively intact pulmonary parenchyma there may be progression to pulmonary fibrosis.
       D. **True.**   These hyaline membranes are a characteristic histological feature of ARDS and are also seen in the respiratory distress syndrome which affects premature babies.
       E. **False.**   Type I pneumocytes are unable to divide. Type II pneumocytes may proliferate to produce alveoli which are lined by cuboidal cells.

14.10 Bronchiectasis:

A. Usually affects the upper lobes of the lungs.

B. Is associated with cystic fibrosis.

C. Is characterised by constriction of bronchi.

D. Is associated with Kartagener's syndrome.

E. May complicate infection with the measles virus.

14.11 Carcinoid tumours of the bronchus:

A. Contain dense-core granules on electron microscopic examination.

B. Usually occur in the periphery of the lung.

C. May produce 5-hydroxytryptamine.

D. Characteristically grow along the alveolar septa.

E. May cause haemoptysis.

14.12 Exposures to the following materials have a proven positive association with carcinoma of the lung:

A. Asbestos.

B. Cigar smoke.

C. Cigarette smoke.

D. Uranium.

E. Radon.

(Answers overleaf)

14.10 A. False. The lower lobes are the most common site of bronchiectasis.

B. True. The hyperviscous mucus in the airways of subjects with cystic fibrosis leads to plugging and secondary bacterial infection.

C. False. Bronchiectasis is characterised by dilation of the affected bronchi.

D. True. Kartagener's syndrome and other syndromes with immotile cilia cause decreased mucociliary clearance of organisms and debris from the lungs.

E. True. A measles pneumonia may lead to a chronic secondary bacterial infection and subsequent bronchiectasis.

14.11 A. True. These dense-core granules are an indication of their neuro-endocrine differentiation.

B. False. The majority of bronchial carcinoids arise around the major central bronchi.

C. True. 5-Hydroxytryptamine (serotonin) is one of the mediators which contribute to the carcinoid syndrome (diarrhoea, flushing, right-sided heart valve lesions).

D. False. This pattern of growth is characteristic of bronchioloalveolar carcinoma. Carcinoid tumours are usually solid nodules which may protrude through the bronchial wall to form 'dumb-bell' tumours.

E. True. The central location of bronchial carcinoids often leads to haemoptysis and obstructive changes in the distal lung.

14.12 A. True. The effect of exposure to asbestos and cigarette smoke is multiplicative rather than additive.

B. True. There is an increased incidence of lung cancer in cigar smokers but it is less than that of cigarette smokers.

C. True. Heavy smokers have a risk of developing lung cancer which is at least 20 times greater than non-smokers.

D. True. Non-smokers who work in uranium mines have an increased risk of developing lung cancer.

E. True. This radioactive gas has been associated with lung cancer. It is present in granite and is present in significant amounts in some British houses.

14.13 Centrilobular emphysema:

A. Is closely associated with cigarette smoking.
B. Is associated with α_1-antitrypsin deficiency.
C. May be complicated by spontaneous pneumothorax.
D. Is most commonly sited in the lower lobes.
E. Is characterised by destruction of elastin in alveolar walls.

14.14 Sarcoidosis:

A. Is caused by proliferation of Langerhans' cells.
B. Is associated with hypogammaglobulinaemia.
C. May produce a diffuse interstitial alveolitis.
D. May be diagnosed using the Schick test.
E. Is characterised histologically by non-caseating granulomas.

14.15 Small-cell carcinomas of the lung:

A. Are not associated with cigarette smoking.
B. Are commoner in men than in women.
C. Have a 5-year survival rate of about 30%.
D. Are usually amenable to surgical resection.
E. Often show nuclear moulding on histological examination.

(Answers overleaf)

14.13 A. True.
   B. False. α_1-Antitrypsin deficiency is associated with a panlobular pattern of emphysema.
   C. True. Bullae may rupture to produce a pneumothorax.
   D. False. Centrilobular emphysema occurs most frequently in the upper lobes, contrasting with panlobular emphysema which usually affects the lower lobes.
   E. True. This is a characteristic feature of all the emphysemas.

14.14 A. False. Histiocytosis X is due to proliferation of Langerhans' cells. Histiocytes (macrophages) are present in sarcoidosis but are a reactive, rather than proliferative, phenomenon.
   B. False. Sarcoidosis is associated with *hyper*gammaglobulinaemia. Other biochemical abnormalities include hypercalcaemia, hypercalcuria and raised serum levels of angiotensin-converting enzyme.
   C. True. Sarcoidosis is one of the many causes of a diffuse interstitial alveolitis. The alveolitis may be severe enough to produce a 'honeycomb' lung.
   D. False. The Schick test is used to demonstrate immunity to diphtheria. The Kveim test, an injection of a suspension of sarcoid material (usually spleen), may be used in the diagnosis of sarcoidosis.
   E. True. Non-caseating granulomas are the histological hallmark but other causes of granulomatous inflammation must be excluded.

14.15 A. False. There is a strong association between cigarette smoking and small-cell carcinoma of the lung.
   B. True.
   C. False. The 5-year survival rate is very low, of the order of 2–3%.
   D. False. Small-cell carcinomas are usually widely invasive and metastasise early, so are not surgically resectable. The firstline treatment is usually chemotherapy.
   E. True. This is a characteristic feature which leads to the alternative name of 'oat-cell' carcinoma.

14.16 Silicosis:

 A. May affect gold miners.
 B. Is caused by silica particles greater than 50 μm in diameter.
 C. Is associated with tuberculosis.
 D. May cause right ventricular hypertrophy.
 E. May cause malignant mesothelioma of the pleura.

14.17 Chronic bronchitis:

 A. Is usually defined as a persistent productive cough for at least 3 consecutive months in at least 2 consecutive years.
 B. Rarely co-exists with emphysema.
 C. Is not associated with cigarette smoking.
 D. Is associated with hypoplasia of mucin-secreting glands.
 E. Is associated with infection by *Haemophilus influenzae*.

14.18 The following conditions can cause pulmonary hypertension:

 A. Wegener's granulomatosis.
 B. Multiple pulmonary emboli.
 C. A right-to-left intracardiac shunt.
 D. Residence at a high altitude.
 E. Transposition of the great vessels.

(Answers overleaf)

14.16 A. **True.**   Other occupations which may result in exposure to silica include copper mining, sandblasting, stonemasons and pottery workers.

B. **False.**   Particles of this diameter are unlikely to reach the alveoli. Particles of about 5 μm in diameter are most likely to cause silicosis.

C. **True.**   Some 10–80% of subjects with silicosis have concomitant tuberculosis.

D. **True.**   Progressive obliteration of the pulmonary vasculature by fibrosis can lead to pulmonary hypertension and right ventricular hypertrophy.

E. **False.**   Asbestosis, not silicosis, is implicated in the causation of malignant mesothelioma.

14.17 A. **True.**   Many people have a productive cough at some time during a year; it is the persistence of a cough that helps to define chronic bronchitis.

B. **False.**   Chronic bronchitis and emphysema are co-existent in the vast majority of subjects.

C. **False.**   Cigarette smoking is thought to be the most important causative agent in chronic bronchitis. Other air pollution, such as sulphur dioxide, is also important.

D. **False.**   *Hyper*plasia of the mucin-secreting glands is an invariable feature of chronic bronchitis. The excessive mucin causes airway plugging.

E. **True.**   Other commonly isolated organisms are coagulase-positive staphylococci.

14.18 A. **True.**   Wegener's granulomatosis can lead to pulmonary hypertension by causing narrowing of arteries in the pulmonary vasculature.

B. **True.**   Multiple pulmonary emboli obstruct the flow of blood through the lungs.

C. **False.**   A right-to-left shunt would decrease blood flow through the lungs and could produce pulmonary hypotension.

D. **True.**   Habitation at high altitude causes chronic hypoxia with vasoconstriction and subsequently pulmonary hypertension.

E. **True.**   In this anomaly there is increased blood flow through the lungs.

14.19 Squamous cell carcinoma of the lung:

    A. Is commoner in females than in males.

    B. Is usually situated in the periphery of the lung.

    C. Rarely metastasises.

    D. Has a 5-year survival rate of about 60%.

    E. Contains cytoplasmic mucin globules.

14.20 A false-negative reaction to the tuberculin test may occur in the following circumstances:

    A. Cyclosporin therapy.

    B. Malignant lymphoma.

    C. Viral infections.

    D. Malnutrition.

    E. Active tuberculosis.

14.21 Hyaline membrane disease (HMD) in neonates (infantile respiratory distress syndrome) is associated with:

    A. Postmaturity.

    B. Delivery by caesarean section.

    C. Birthweight of more than 4.5 kg.

    D. A deficiency of pulmonary surfactant.

    E. Maternal diabetes mellitus.

(Answers overleaf)

14.19 A. False. Squamous cell carcinoma of the lung is commoner in males than in females.
   B. False. Squamous cell carcinomas usually arise centrally in a major bronchus; adenocarcinomas tend to occur in the periphery.
   C. False. About 50% of subjects with squamous cell carcinoma of the lung have metastatic disease at presentation.
   D. False. The overall 5-year survival rate is only 5–10%.
   E. False. Adenocarcinomas contain intracytoplasmic mucin. Squamous cell carcinomas reveal their differentiation by production of keratin and intercellular bridges.

14.20 A. True. Cyclosporin is an immunosuppressant drug often used to prevent rejection of allografts. The reduction in cell-mediated immunity may cause a false-negative tuberculin test.
   B. True. Malignant lymphoma may produce a deficiency in cell-mediated immunity.
   C. True. Cell-mediated immunity may be depressed in certain viral infections (e.g. HIV infection).
   D. True. Immune paresis occurs in malnutrition.
   E. True. An overwhelming tuberculous infection may cause a false-negative tuberculin test, a fact of considerable clinical importance.

14.21 A. False. HMD is most common in premature infants of less than 36 weeks' gestation.
   B. True. There is a higher incidence of HMD in babies delivered by caesarean section. It is postulated that vaginal delivery may assist respiration by forcing fluid from the lungs by mechanical pressure.
   C. False. HMD is associated with a birthweight of less than 4.5 kg.
   D. True. This deficiency is one of the basic mechanisms causing HMD by preventing lung expansion.
   E. True. The reason for this association is not clear.

14.22 Pulmonary adenochondroma:

A. Is regarded as an autonomous neoplasm.
B. May present as a 'coin' lesion on chest radiograph.
C. Has poorly-defined borders.
D. Is usually a central lesion.
E. Must always be surgically removed.

14.23 The following are viruses which commonly cause rhinitis:

A. Coronaviruses.
B. Rhinoviruses.
C. Cytomegalovirus.
D. *Haemophilus influenzae.*
E. Echoviruses.

14.24 Squamous cell carcinoma of the nasal passages and sinuses:

A. Is associated with working in the wood and furniture industries.
B. Is associated with infection by Epstein–Barr virus.
C. Is commoner in Europe than in the Far East.
D. May produce keratin.
E. May have an associated lymphoid infiltrate.

(Answers overleaf)

14.22 A. False. Pulmonary adenochondromas are thought to be hamartomas; their growth ceases after puberty, so that they appear to be under normal mechanisms of growth control.
   B. True. They are often an incidental finding on chest radiograph.
   C. False. The borders are usually sharply defined.
   D. False. Pulmonary adenochondromas usually occur in the peripheral parts of the lung.
   E. False. They are often removed because a histological diagnosis is required to differentiate them from other lung tumours, but if a diagnosis can be made without removal then they can be left in situ.

14.23 A. True.
   B. True. These viruses are the most common cause of rhinitis.
   C. False. Cytomegalovirus rarely, if ever, causes a rhinitis.
   D. False. *Haemophilus influenzae* is a bacterium.
   E. True.

14.24 A. False. Adenocarcinoma of the nasal passage and sinuses is associated with woodworking.
   B. True. EBV genome may be isolated from these tumours.
   C. False. This tumour is more common in China and the Far East than in Europe.
   D. True. The well-differentiated variants may produce keratin.
   E. True. This lymphoid infiltrate was so prominent in some tumours that they were mislabelled as 'lymphoepitheliomas'.

15

Alimentary system

15.1 Oral leukoplakia:
A. Is not associated with cigarette smoking.
B. Has a higher incidence in India and Sri Lanka than in Europe.
C. Is characterised by hyperkeratosis when examined histologically.
D. Can be a premalignant condition.
E. Is not associated with excessive alcohol consumption.

15.2 Carcinomas of the anus and anal canal:
A. May be of squamous cell type.
B. May be of adenocarcinomatous type.
C. Have a higher incidence in promiscuous homosexual males.
D. Are associated with condyloma acuminata.
E. Rarely metastasise to the inguinal lymph nodes.

15.3 Primary gastric lymphomas:
A. Are the rarest intestinal lymphomas.
B. Are usually of T-cell type.
C. Have a 5-year survival rate of 5% if confined to the stomach.
D. Usually arise from the mucosa-associated lymphoid tissue.
E. Are rarely of Hodgkin's type.

15.1 **A. False.** Leukoplakia is associated with heavy cigarette smoking.
  B. True. This is attributed to the chewing of betel quids in India and Sri Lanka.
  C. True. This is the feature which gives leukoplakia its white appearance.
  D. True. The squamous epithelium in leukoplakia may show dysplasia, as well as hyperkeratosis, and so may herald the onset of squamous cell carcinoma.
  E. False. Leukoplakia is associated with high alcohol consumption (poor oral hygiene is another association).

15.2 **A. True.** Those carcinomas which arise in the lower part of the anal canal are usually squamous cell carcinomas.
  B. True. Carcinomas rising in the upper part of the anal canal, above the dentate line, show adenocarcinomatous differentiation.
  C. True. This may be due to acquisition of viral infections, particularly human papillomaviruses.
  D. True. The association between anal squamous cell carcinomas and human papillomavirus infection appears to be analogous with the situation seen in the cervix uteri.
  E. False. The inguinal and lateral pelvic lymph nodes are common sites for metastasis.

15.3 **A. False.** The stomach is the most common site for lymphoma in the alimentary tract; 40% of primary gastrointestinal lymphomas arise there.
  B. False. Gastric lymphomas are usually of non-Hodgkin's B-cell type.
  C. False. The 5-year survival rate for lymphomas confined to the stomach is about 50%; the prognosis is much worse if regional lymph nodes are involved.
  D. True. This is why they are usually of B-cell origin.
  E. True. Primary Hodgkin's disease of the gastrointestinal tract is vanishingly rare.

15.4 *Helicobacter pylori*:

    A. Is a Gram-positive organism.

    B. Is associated with active chronic gastritis.

    C. Is more often found in the body than in the antrum of the stomach.

    D. Activates complement by the alternative pathway.

    E. Colonises normal small intestinal mucosa.

15.5 **The following conditions may arise as complications of appendicitis:**

    A. Subphrenic abscess.

    B. Mucocele of the appendix.

    C. Portal pylephlebitis.

    D. Peritonitis.

    E. Carcinoma of the appendix.

15.6 **Coeliac disease (gluten enteropathy):**

    A. Is characterised histologically by villous atrophy and increased numbers of intraepithelial lymphocytes.

    B. Is associated with an increased risk of developing intestinal lymphoma.

    C. Is associated with the HLA haplotype B8.

    D. Is associated with dermatitis herpetiformis.

    E. Usually responds to broad-spectrum antibiotics.

(Answers overleaf)

15.4 **A.** **False.** *Helicobacter pylori* is a Gram-negative organism.
B. **True.** Some 90% of biopsies with active chronic gastritis contain *Helicobacter*-like organisms.
C. **False.** It is found most commonly in the antrum.
D. **True.** This activation of complement initiates the inflammatory response.
E. **False.** Normal small intestinal mucosa is not colonised but, interestingly, *Helicobacter pylori* may be found in the heterotopic gastric mucosa of a Meckel's diverticulum.

15.5 **A.** **True.** Pus from a perforated appendix may track up the paracolic gutter and form a subphrenic collection.
B. **True.** If focal inflammation of the base of the appendix causes fibrous stenosis of the lumen then mucous secretions may dilate the appendiceal tip to produce a mucocele.
C. **True.** Extension of infected thrombus up the portal vein can lead to a portal pylephlebitis.
D. **True.** Perforation of an inflamed appendix can lead to a generalised peritonitis.
E. **False.** Carcinoma of the appendix has not been shown to arise as a complication of appendicitis. It may however be present in an inflamed appendix and may have initiated the inflammatory process by obstructing the lumen or eroding through the wall.

15.6 **A.** **True.** These are the characteristic histological appearances.
B. **True.** Intestinal lymphoma occurs in a significant number of subjects with untreated coeliac disease.
C. **True.** It is also associated with DW3.
D. **True.**
E. **False.** Coeliac disease responds to a gluten-free diet. Tropical sprue and Whipple's disease are malabsorptive conditions which may improve with antibiotic therapy.

15.7   Carcinoid tumours of the small bowel:
  A.   React positively with argentaffin stains.
  B.   Often produce 5-hydroxytryptamine (serotonin).
  C.   Never metastasise.
  D.   Usually arise in the ileum.
  E.   May produce smooth-muscle proliferation within the endocardium.

15.8   Crohn's disease:
  A.   Occurs most frequently in the ileum.
  B.   Is characterised histologically by diffuse superficial inflammation.
  C.   May cause intestinal obstruction.
  D.   Often produces granulomas in the bowel and lymph nodes.
  E.   Usually presents after the age of 40 years.

15.9   Peptic duodenal ulcers:
  A.   Are less common than gastric peptic ulcers.
  B.   Are associated with hyposecretion of gastric acid.
  C.   Are usually multiple.
  D.   Are usually sited in the second and third parts of the duodenum.
  E.   Usually require surgical treatment.

(Answers overleaf)

15.7   **A.**   **True.**   Carcinoid tumours usually react with both argentaffin and argyrophil stains.

      B.   **True.**   They also produce prostaglandins, histamine and other mediators of inflammation. It is thought that these are the cause of the flushing and diarrhoea which occur in the carcinoid syndrome.

      C.   **False.**   Metastasis to the liver is quite common.

      D.   **True.**   The ileum is the most common site followed by the jejunum and distal duodenum.

      E.   **True.**   This is thought to result from bradykinin stimulation of mesenchymal cells which undergo differentiation to muscle cells.

15.8   **A.**   **True.**   Although the disease may affect any part of the gastrointestinal system, from mouth to anus, the ileum is most frequently involved.

      B.   **False.**   The inflammation in Crohn's disease is characteristically patchy and involves the full thickness of the bowel wall.

      C.   **True.**   Fibrosis of the bowel wall may cause stenosis and intestinal obstruction.

      D.   **True.**   Granulomas are an important feature in the histological diagnosis of Crohn's disease.

      E.   **False.**   Some 90% of cases present between the ages of 10 and 40 years, but the disease may occur at any age.

15.9   **A.**   **False.**   Duodenal peptic ulcers are still more common than those in the stomach but their relative incidence is declining.

      B.   **False.**   Duodenal peptic ulcers are almost always associated with *hyper*secretion of gastric acid.

      C.   **False.**   They are usually solitary. Multiple ulcers should arouse suspicion of disorders like the Zollinger–Ellison syndrome.

      D.   **False.**   They are usually situated in the first part of the duodenum within 2 cm of the pylorus.

      E.   **False.**   Medical treatments, such as H_2 receptor antagonists, are very effective, and only about 20% of duodenal peptic ulcers require surgical therapy.

15.10 Pyloric stenosis in children:
A. Usually presents after the age of 6 months.
B. Is commoner in female than in male infants.
C. Is characterised by atrophy of the pyloric muscle.
D. Has an incidence of about 4 in 1000 live births in Europe.
E. Is associated with low birthweight.

15.11 Whipple's disease:
A. Is characterised by numerous neutrophils in the lamina propria of the bowel.
B. Is restricted to the bowel.
C. Occurs most frequently in young women.
D. Is a self-limiting disorder.
E. May be diagnosed by electron microscopy of bowel biopsies.

15.12 Meckel's diverticulum:
A. Results from persistence of the proximal part of the vitelline duct.
B. May produce ileal ulceration.
C. Usually occurs in the proximal part of the small bowel.
D. May produce clinical signs mimicking acute appendicitis.
E. May contain heterotopic pancreatic elements.

(Answers overleaf)

15.10 A. False. Presentation, with projectile vomiting, is usually within the first three months of life.
B. False. It is about four times more common in males than in females.
C. False. The pyloric muscle is hypertrophied.
D. True.
E. False. Hypertrophic pyloric stenosis is associated with a higher-than-average birthweight and with babies born to professional parents.

15.11 A. False. The characteristic light-microscopic appearance is of numerous macrophages packed into the lamina propria and submucosa.
B. False. The disease may affect many organs, including lymph nodes, spleen, heart and joints.
C. False. Whipple's disease occurs almost exclusively in middle-aged Caucasian males.
D. False. Without treatment most cases die within a few years. Treatment with antibiotics may result in a rapid recovery.
E. True. Typical bacilliform bodies (*Tropheryma whippelii*) may be seen on electron microscopy.

15.12 A. True. Persistence of the whole of the vitelline duct produces an enteroumbilical fistula.
B. True. Some Meckel's diverticula contain acid-producing ectopic gastric mucosa which can lead to ulceration of distal small bowel.
C. False. Meckel's diverticula usually occur in the distal 80 cm of the ileum.
D. True. If a Meckel's diverticulum becomes inflamed it may produce symptoms and signs similar to those found in acute appendicitis.
E. True.

15.13 Oropharyngeal carcinoma:
  A. Occurs most commonly on the lip.
  B. On the tongue, has a better prognosis if it arises in the posterior, rather than the anterior, half.
  C. Is associated with tobacco chewing.
  D. Is more common in females than males.
  E. Metastasises predominantly by the haematogenous route.

15.14 Carcinoma of the oesophagus:
  A. Is associated with oesophageal achalasia.
  B. Is rare in Iran.
  C. When confined to the wall of the oesophagus, has a 5-year survival rate of about 75%.
  D. Is not associated with cigarette smoking.
  E. Usually arises in the upper third of the oesophagus.

15.15 Ulcerative colitis:
  A. Most often affects the rectum and sigmoid colon.
  B. On histological examination usually exhibits transmural inflammation.
  C. Is not associated with an increased risk of developing colonic carcinoma.
  D. Is associated with erythema nodosum.
  E. May cause Paneth cell hyperplasia.

(Answers overleaf)

15.13 A. True. Some 45% of oropharyngeal carcinomas occur on the lip.
   B. False. The prognosis is better if the tumour occurs on the anterior half of the tongue.
   C. True. It is also associated with other forms of tobacco consumption.
   D. False. Oropharyngeal carcinoma is much more frequent in males, but the incidence amongst females is rising.
   E. False. The predominant route of spread is lymphatic. The retropharyngeal and cervical lymph nodes are the earliest sites of metastases.

15.14 A. True. It is also associated with oesophageal webs and diverticula.
   B. False. The incidence of oesophageal carcinoma in north-eastern Iran is about 300 times greater than that in Britain.
   C. True. If the tumour extends beyond the wall then the prognosis is much worse, with a 5-year survival rate of about 5%.
   D. False. Cigarette smoking and alcohol abuse are both associated with an increased risk of developing oesophageal carcinoma.
   E. False. Approximately 10–15% of oesophageal carcinomas arise in the upper third of the oesophagus. About 50% are located in the middle third and the rest in the lower part of the oesophagus.

15.15 A. True. This is the most common site, and the disease may extend in continuity to involve the whole colon. Isolated right-sided disease may occur but is less common.
   B. False. The inflammation in ulcerative colitis is characteristically confined to the bowel mucosa. Transmural inflammation is a feature of Crohn's disease.
   C. False. There is a considerable risk of developing colonic carcinoma in severe ulcerative colitis of long standing (10 years or more). In such cases, follow-up by colonoscopy and biopsy is required to identify the dysplasia which may precede invasive carcinoma.
   D. True. It may also be associated with pyoderma gangrenosum.
   E. True. In chronic ulcerative colitis there is often a proliferation of Paneth cells at the base of the crypts.

15.16 Carcinoma of the large intestine:

A. Is most frequently sited in the caecum.
B. Has a positive association with familial polyposis coli.
C. Is usually of squamous differentiation.
D. Is commoner in Africa than in Europe.
E. May cause intestinal obstruction.

15.17 Gastric carcinoma:

A. Confined to the mucosa and submucosa, has a treated 5-year survival rate of about 90%.
B. May produce Krukenberg tumours in the ovaries.
C. Is surgically resectable in over 80% of cases.
D. Has a positive association with peptic duodenal ulcer.
E. Is usually of adenocarcinomatous differentiation.

15.18 The following polyps in the large bowel are precancerous:

A. Tubular adenomas.
B. Hamartomatous polyps.
C. Villous adenomas.
D. Metaplastic polyps.
E. Lymphoid polyposis.

(Answers overleaf)

15.16 A. False. The rectum is the commonest site.
   B. True. If familial polyposis coli is not treated by complete colectomy then carcinoma invariably ensues.
   C. False. Almost all carcinomas of the large intestine are adenocarcinomas.
   D. False. Carcinoma of the large intestine is much commoner in Europe than in Africa. Increased gut transit time, due to low-fibre diets, has been proposed as an explanation for this difference.
   E. True. This is most common in left-sided lesions where the intestinal contents are more solid.

15.17 A. True. These tumours are usually called 'early' gastric cancers and have a good prognosis even in the presence of local nodal metastases.
   B. True. Krukenberg tumours consist of metastatic adenocarcinoma cells set in a desmoplastic stroma.
   C. False. Only about 45% of gastric carcinomas are amenable to surgical resection at their time of presentation.
   D. False. There is a small positive association with peptic gastric ulcers but no positive, and possibly a negative, association with peptic duodenal ulcers.
   E. True. The vast majority of gastric cancers are adenocarcinomas.

15.18 A. True. Tubular adenomas show varying degrees of epithelial dysplasia, and carcinomas have been shown to arise within such adenomas.
   B. False. Hamartomatous polyps are still under the normal mechanisms of growth control.
   C. True. Villous adenomas are more likely to progress to carcinoma than are tubular adenomas.
   D. False. Metaplastic polyps are a frequent finding in adult colons. Carcinomas have not been shown to arise from them at a frequency above that of the background colon.
   E. False. In this condition subepithelial collections of lymphocytes produce a polypoid appearance.

15.19 Cholera:
   A. Is usually accompanied by marked mucosal inflammation and ulceration of the intestine.
   B. Is caused by infection with *Shigella sonnei*.
   C. May cause death from dehydration and electrolyte imbalance.
   D. Is caused by a toxin which reduces adenylate cyclase activity.
   E. Is usually transmitted by contaminated water supplies.

15.20 Hirschsprung's disease:
   A. Usually affects the right side of the colon.
   B. Has a positive association with necrotising enterocolitis.
   C. Is caused by a failure of migration of neuroblasts.
   D. May cause chronic constipation.
   E. Is associated with cystic fibrosis.

15.21 In Dukes' system of staging rectal carcinomas:
   A. Stage B indicates involvement of lymph nodes close to the bowel.
   B. Stage A indicates that the tumour has not penetrated the muscularis mucosae.
   C. Stage C has a 5-year survival rate of about 30%.
   D. Stage B has a 5-year survival rate of about 50%.
   E. Stage A has a 5-year survival rate of about 90%.

(Answers overleaf)

15.19 A. False. The diarrhoea of cholera is caused by the action of a toxin; the mucosa is not actually invaded by the bacteria, so that mucosal inflammation is slight and there is no ulceration.
  B. False. Shigellae cause bacillary dysentery. Cholera is caused by *Vibrio cholerae*.
  C. True. The watery diarrhoea may be so extreme that death from these causes may occur.
  D. False. The toxin *increases* the activity of adenylate cyclase.
  E. True.

15.20 A. False. Hirschsprung's disease affects the distal rectum and colon with a variable extension proximally.
  B. True. Necrotising enterocolitis is the commonest cause of death in Hirschsprung's disease.
  C. True. The neuroblasts fail to migrate from the vagus, so intramural parasympathetic nerve plexuses fail to develop.
  D. True. Chronic constipation is the usual presentation of the mild form of Hirschsprung's disease.
  E. False. Intestinal obstruction may occur in neonates with cystic fibrosis but this is due to meconium ileus. There is no positive association between Hirschsprung's disease and cystic fibrosis.

15.21 A. False. Lymph node involvement puts a tumour into stage C.
  B. False. Stage A indicates that the tumour has not penetrated the muscularis propria. If the muscularis mucosae has not been breached then the tumour is not regarded as invasive and the terms 'severe epithelial dysplasia' or 'intramucosal carcinoma' may be used.
  C. True. The prognosis is worst for cases where the lymph nodes at the mesenteric resection margin are involved.
  D. False. The 5-year survival rate is about 80%.
  E. True. Patients with stage A disease can be reassured of the excellent prognosis following resection.

15.22 The following may occur as benign polyps of the large intestine:

A. Kaposi's sarcoma.
B. Lipomas.
C. Haemangiosarcomas.
D. Peutz–Jeghers polyps.
E. Leiomyomas.

15.23 Diverticular disease of the colon:

A. Is associated with high-fibre diets.
B. Is associated with atrophy of the muscles of the bowel wall.
C. Is usually situated in the ascending colon.
D. May cause vesico-colic fistulae.
E. Is associated with an increased risk of developing colonic carcinoma.

15.24 Gastric carcinoma:

A. Is associated with hyperchlorhydria.
B. Is less common in Japan than in Britain.
C. Has an increased incidence in people with pernicious anaemia.
D. Has a peak incidence in the fourth decade of life.
E. Has been increasing in incidence in Britain since 1960.

(Answers overleaf)

15.22 A. False. Kaposi's sarcoma can produce polypoid lesions in the large intestine but it is a malignant tumour of vascular differentiation.

B. True. Submucosal lipomas may produce a polypoid appearance.

C. False. Haemangiosarcomas are a very rare cause of polypoid lesions in the large intestine, but, like Kaposi's sarcoma, they are malignant, rather than benign, tumours.

D. True. The polyps which occur in Peutz–Jeghers syndrome may occur anywhere in the intestine.

E. True. Benign tumours of the muscularis mucosae and muscularis propria may produce polypoid lesions in the large intestine.

15.23 A. False. Diverticular disease is associated with low-fibre diets.

B. False. The muscles of the bowel wall are hypertrophied.

C. False. The diverticula are found most frequently in the sigmoid colon.

D. True. This may lead to the dramatic symptom of pneumaturia.

E. False. There is no evidence that diverticular disease is directly associated with colonic carcinoma although there is a similar geographical distribution which may be related to low-fibre diets. Diverticular disease may be confused with carcinoma on macroscopic examination when there has been chronic inflammation and fibrosis.

15.24 A. False. Gastric carcinoma is accompanied by *hypo*chlorhydria in about 80% of cases.

B. False. Gastric carcinoma has a much higher incidence in Japan than in Britain.

C. True. Gastric carcinoma also has an increased incidence in people with atrophic gastritis. In both instances the increase is statistically valid but not great enough to justify screening of these populations.

D. False. Most cases of gastric carcinoma present in people over the age of 50 years.

E. False. The incidence in Britain has been decreasing in recent years but the reasons for this are not clear.

15.25 Familial adenomatous polyposis:
- **A.** Is transmitted as an autosomal recessive condition.
- **B.** Has been localised to a gene on the short arm of chromosome 6.
- **C.** Affects males more commonly than females.
- **D.** Rarely progresses to carcinoma before the age of 35 years.
- **E.** Is characterised by adenomas sited exclusively in the large intestine.

15.26 The following hepatic conditions have a positive association with ulcerative colitis:
- **A.** Chronic active hepatitis.
- **B.** Chronic pericholangitis.
- **C.** Sclerosing cholangitis.
- **D.** Cirrhosis.
- **E.** Fatty change (steatosis).

15.27 The following are bacterial causes of intestinal infection:
- **A.** *Giardia lamblia.*
- **B.** *Balantidium coli.*
- **C.** *Schistosoma mansoni.*
- **D.** *Escherichia coli.*
- **E.** *Histoplasma capsulatum.*

15.28 Gonococcal proctitis:
- **A.** Is typically characterised by a chronic inflammatory response.
- **B.** May be transmitted by anal intercourse.
- **C.** Is caused by a Gram-positive diplococcus.
- **D.** Is thought to be an aetiological agent for anal carcinoma.
- **E.** Is often preceded by broad-spectrum antibiotic therapy.

(Answers overleaf)

15.25 A. False. It follows an autosomal dominant pattern of inheritance.
   B. False. The gene has been localised to the long arm of chromosome 5.
   C. False. The sexes are affected equally because it is a Mendelian autosomal condition.
   D. False. Progression to carcinoma almost always occurs before the age of 35 years.
   E. False. Adenomas also occur in the small intestine.

15.26 A. True. There is an increased prevalence of chronic active hepatitis in subjects with ulcerative colitis.
   B. True. Chronic inflammation centred around bile ducts, chronic pericholangitis, is seen in ulcerative colitis and is thought to be a precursor of sclerosing cholangitis.
   C. True.
   D. True. Sclerosing cholangitis and chronic active hepatitis can both progress to a hepatic cirrhosis.
   E. True. This fatty change may be due to protein deficiency, anaemia and infection.

15.27 A. False. *Giardia* is a flagellate protozoan. It is a cause of 'traveller's diarrhoea' and may produce a malabsorptive state.
   B. False. This ciliated protozoan produces intestinal infection in tropical and sub-tropical countries.
   C. False. Schistosomes are members of the fluke family.
   D. True. Enterotoxic strains of *Escherichia coli* may cause diarrhoea, especially in neonates.
   E. False. *Histoplasma capsulatum* is a fungus.

15.28 A. False. The inflammatory response is typically an acute exudative pattern.
   B. True. Genito-anal spread may occur in females, but in males it is mainly transmitted by anal intercourse and is included within the 'gay bowel' syndrome.
   C. False. The gonococcus is a Gram-negative organism.
   D. False. The increased incidence of anal carcinoma in promiscuous male homosexuals is thought to have an infective origin but the aetiological agent is thought to be the human papillomavirus.
   E. False. Pseudomembranous colitis is caused by overgrowth of *Clostridium difficile* following administration of broad-spectrum antibiotics.

15.29 Intestinal tuberculosis:

   A. Usually occurs in the large intestine.

   B. Has decreased in incidence with the pasteurisation of milk.

   C. May lead to stricture formation.

   D. Produces a histological picture easily distinguished from Crohn's disease.

   E. May occur as a complication of pulmonary tuberculosis.

15.30 Intestinal actinomycosis:

   A. Is caused by an organism which is a normal oral commensal.

   B. Affects the duodenum most frequently.

   C. May produce macroscopically visible 'sulphur granules'.

   D. Usually has a short duration.

   E. May be complicated by sinus formation.

(Answers overleaf)

15.29 A. False. Tuberculosis is almost entirely confined to the small intestine.

B. True. Pasteurisation of milk and tuberculin testing of cattle has dramatically reduced the incidence of bovine tuberculosis in Britain.

C. True. Other complications include perforation of tuberculous ulcers and malabsorption due to loss of mucosal surface area or lymphatic blockage.

D. False. The histological appearances of tuberculosis and Crohn's disease are virtually identical.

E. True. Intestinal infection may occur after the swallowing of infected sputum.

15.30 A. True. *Actinomyces israelii* is a normal commensal of the mouth which has the ability to resist acid digestion.

B. False. The caecum and appendix are the sites which are most commonly affected.

C. True. These are colonies of the organism.

D. False. The illness typically has a protracted chronic course.

E. True. Fistulae may also occur.

16

Liver, biliary system and exocrine pancreas

16.1 Gallstones:

A. Of pure cholesterol type are the most frequent.
B. Of pigment type are usually solitary.
C. May lead to formation of a mucocele.
D. Of mixed type are usually laminated in cross-section.
E. May cause pancreatitis.

16.2 Fatty change in the liver (steatosis) has an increased incidence in these groups of people:

A. Alcoholics.
B. Obese people.
C. People with a jejunoileal bypass.
D. Subjects with diabetes mellitus.
E. Subjects on total parenteral nutrition.

16.3 α_1-Antitrypsin deficiency:

A. Is due to a failure of the liver to secrete copper into bile.
B. May lead to hepatic cirrhosis.
C. Is characterised histologically by hyaline intracytoplasmic globules.
D. Is associated with pulmonary emphysema.
E. May be diagnosed by histology alone.

(Answers overleaf)

16.1 **A.** **False.** Mixed stones are the most frequent. Pure cholesterol stones account for about 10% of all gallstones.
  B. **False.** Pigment type stones are almost always multiple.
  C. **True.** A gallstone which impacts in the cystic duct can lead to mucocele formation.
  D. **True.** This is the characteristic macroscopic appearance.
  E. **True.** Gallstones may enter the common bile duct and lodge at the ampulla of Vater causing an obstructive pancreatitis.

16.2 **A.** **True.** Liver biopsies from alcoholics show fatty change in approximately 40% of cases.
  B. **True.** Fatty change in the liver is a common accompaniment of obesity.
  C. **True.** Non-alcoholic steatohepatitis, with progression to cirrhosis, can occur in this condition as well as simple fatty change.
  D. **True.** There is an increased incidence of steatosis in subjects with diabetes mellitus.
  E. **True.** The reason for this is not clear.

16.3 **A.** **False.** α_1-Antitrypsin deficiency is due to defective synthesis of α_1-antitrypsin. Wilson's disease is due to failure of the liver to excrete copper into bile.
  B. **True.** Hepatic disease occurs in at least two-thirds of subjects with α_1-antitrypsin deficiency.
  C. **True.** Similar globules may be seen in other diseases which affect the liver, so the appearances are not totally specific.
  D. **True.**
  E. **False.** Since the PAS-positive globules and the pattern of liver disease are not totally specific, the diagnosis should be confirmed by phenotypic evaluation of the α_1-antitrypsin.

16.4   Liver cell carcinoma (hepatocellular carcinoma):

   A.   Is more common in Europe than in Southern Africa.
   B.   Is more common in females than in males.
   C.   Is often associated with raised serum levels of
         α-fetoprotein.
   D.   Is associated with hepatic cirrhosis.
   E.   Is associated with hepatitis B surface antigenaemia.

16.5   Carcinoma of the pancreas: *adenocarcinomas*

   A.   Is usually of squamous cell type.
   B.   Has a positive association with cigarette smoking.
   C.   Has a positive association with venous thromboses.
   D.   Decreased in incidence in Britain in the late 20th century.
   E.   Often causes a patient to present with weight loss.

16.6   Chronic cholecystitis:

   A.   Is characterised histologically by fibrosis and
         Aschoff–Rokitansky sinuses.
   B.   Is more common in males than in females.
   C.   Is associated with cholelithiasis in 50% of cases.
   D.   Is associated with a culture-positive bacterial infection in
         less than 30% of cases.
   E.   May cause dystrophic calcification.

(Answers overleaf)

16.4 **A. False.** Hepatocellular carcinoma has a striking geographical distribution with a high incidence south of the Sahara in Africa and in Southeast Asia.
B. False. Hepatocellular carcinoma is commoner in males than in females.
C. True. α-Fetoprotein is not a totally specific or sensitive marker for hepatocellular carcinoma but it is raised in about 60–70% of cases.
D. True. Some 60–80% of subjects with hepatocellular carcinoma have hepatic cirrhosis.
E. True. About 50% of subjects with hepatocellular carcinoma have a hepatitis B surface antigenaemia.

16.5 **A. False.** The majority of pancreatic carcinomas are adenocarcinomas.
B. True. It is also associated with diabetes mellitus.
C. True. This is Trousseau's sign.
D. False. The incidence is increasing in Britain; at present there are about 6000 cases per year.
E. True. The signs and symptoms of pancreatic carcinoma are often not specific because its location does not produce many localising signs (except obstructive jaundice if it occurs at the head of the pancreas). This lack of specific signs leads to late presentation and a dismal overall prognosis.

16.6 **A. True.** These, and an infiltrate of chronic inflammatory cells, are the characteristic histological findings.
B. False. Chronic cholecystitis is more common in females than in males by a ratio of 3:1.
C. False. Gallstones are present in virtually all cases of chronic cholecystitis.
D. True. Bacterial infection does not appear to play a role in all cases of chronic cholecystitis.
E. True. Chronic cholecystitis may produce a 'porcelain' gallbladder.

16.7 **In viral hepatitis A:**

- **A.** A carrier state is common following initial infection.
- **B.** The mortality rate is about 10%.
- **C.** Infection is transmitted mainly by the parenteral route.
- **D.** The incubation period is 2–4 weeks.
- **E.** The infective units are called Dane particles. *Hep B*

16.8 **Carcinoma of the gallbladder:**

- **A.** Has a 5-year survival rate of about 40%.
- **B.** Is commoner in men than in women.
- **C.** Is asymptomatic in about 25% of cases.
- **D.** Has a positive association with gallstones.
- **E.** Has a peak incidence in the fourth decade.

16.9 **The following are risk factors for formation of cholesterol stones in the gallbladder:**

- **A.** Obesity. *T*
- **B.** Chronic haemolytic anaemia. *— pigment stones - bilirubin*
- **C.** Ileal bypass. *T*
- **D.** Alcoholic hepatic cirrhosis. *mu [...] pigment*
- **E.** Clofibrate therapy. *T* *stone*

↑ plasma cholesterol level

↑ biliary secretion of cholesterol

(Answers overleaf)

16.7   **A.**   **False.**   A carrier state does not exist.
B.   **False.**   The mortality rate is about 0.1%.
C.   **False.**   The majority of cases arise from the orofaecal route of transmission. Parenteral transmission is rare because no carrier state exists.
D.   **True.**
E.   **False.**   Dane particles are the infectious units of hepatitis B.

16.8   **A.**   **False.**   The average 5-year survival rate is only 3%.
B.   **False.**   Carcinoma of the gallbladder is twice as frequent in women as in men.
C.   **True.**   About one-quarter of cases are incidental findings at laparotomy or cholecystectomy.
D.   **True.**   Gallstones are present in at least 75% of cases of carcinoma compared with about 10% of the general population.
E.   **False.**   The incidence rises to a peak in the seventh decade in women and in the eighth decade in men.

16.9   **A.**   **True.**   There is increased hepatic secretion of cholesterol in obese individuals.
B.   **False.**   Chronic haemolysis is a risk factor for the formation of pigment stones in the gallbladder.
C.   **True.**
D.   **False.**   Alcoholic hepatic cirrhosis is a risk factor for pigment stones; the reason for this is not known.
E.   **True.**   Clofibrate reduces plasma cholesterol levels but increases biliary secretion of cholesterol.

16.10 The following are features of portal hypertension:

A. Oesophageal varices.
B. Ascites.
C. Rectal varices.
D. Splenic atrophy.
E. 'Caput medusa' of the anterior abdominal wall.

16.11 Hepatitis C virus:

A. Is spread predominantly by the orofaecal route.
B. Is the commonest cause of post-transfusional hepatitis.
C. May cause hepatic cirrhosis.
D. Is a defective RNA virus.
E. Usually produces a well-defined symptomatic illness.

often asymptomatic

(Answers overleaf)

16.10 A. True. In portal hypertension there is enlargement of portosystemic anastomoses. At the lower oesophagus there are anastomoses between the left gastric vein of the portal system and the azygos minor vein of the systemic circulation.

B. True. Increased hydrostatic pressure in the portal system encourages the formation of ascitic fluid.

C. True. In the rectum there is a portosystemic anastomosis between the superior haemorrhoidal veins of the portal system and the middle and inferior haemorrhoidal veins of the systemic system.

D. False. There is splenomegaly due to congestion of the spleen. There may be subsequent hypersplenism with anaemia and thrombocytopenia.

E. True. The 'caput medusa' is formed by dilation of the paraumbilical veins due to their connection with the branches of the portal vein in the falciform ligament.

16.11 A. False. Hepatitis C virus is spread predominantly by the parenteral route and possibly venereally. Hepatitis A virus is spread by the orofaecal route.

B. True. The incidence of hepatitis B after blood transfusion has decreased with the advent of screening donor blood. Hepatitis C is now the commonest cause of hepatitis after blood transfusion or the administration of blood products.

C. True. Hepatitis C infection may become chronic and lead to hepatic cirrhosis.

D. False. Delta agent is a defective RNA virus which requires the presence of hepatitis B virus to complete its infective cycle.

E. False. Hepatitis C infection often passes without being noticed, but despite this it can lead to chronic liver disease.

16.12 Primary biliary cirrhosis:
   A. Affects males more often than females.
   B. Is associated with chronic inflammatory bowel disease.
   C. Is associated with anti-mitochondrial auto-antibodies.
   D. May lead to copper accumulation in the liver.
   E. Is characterised histologically by bile duct destruction.

16.13 Liver cell adenomas: *benign*
   A. Are malignant tumours.
   B. May cause haemoperitoneum.
   C. Have a positive association with taking anabolic or
   oestrogenic steroids.
   D. May cause hepatomegaly.
   E. Are of vascular origin.   *hepatocytes origin*

16.14 Acute pancreatitis:
   A. May be due to infection with the mumps virus. T
   B. May be diagnosed by measurement of serum amylase. T
   C. Often causes hypercalcaemia. F, hypo
   D. Is more common in children than in adults. F
   E. May be due to acute alcohol intoxication. T

16.15 Jaundice:
   A. Is usually observable when serum bilirubin concentration
   exceeds 40 µmol/l. T
   B. May cause kernicterus in the newborn.
   C. Is due to predominantly unconjugated bilirubin in
   Dubin–Johnson syndrome.
   D. May be due to hereditary spherocytosis.
   E. May be due to congenital metabolic defects.

(Answers overleaf)

16.12 A. False. Females are affected much more commonly than are males.
   B. False. Sclerosing cholangitis is associated with chronic inflammatory bowel disease, particularly ulcerative colitis, but there is no such association with primary biliary cirrhosis.
   C. True. The presence of these antibodies is an important diagnostic feature.
   D. True. Copper accumulates because it can no longer be excreted adequately in the bile.
   E. True. This bile duct destruction may be accompanied by granuloma formation.

16.13 A. False. As their name implies, liver cell adenomas are benign tumours.
   B. True. Liver cell adenomas may rupture, leading to bleeding into the peritoneal cavity, but this is an uncommon event.
   C. True. They may also arise spontaneously.
   D. True.
   E. False. Liver cell adenomas are benign tumours of hepatocytic origin. Angiomas, derived from vascular cells, may also occur in the liver.

16.14 A. True. Other causes include obstruction of the pancreatic duct, bile reflux, hyperparathyroidism and hypothermia.
   B. True. The serum amylase is initially greatly elevated.
   C. False. *Hypo*calcaemia may occur due to the consumption of calcium in the abdominal fat necrosis.
   D. False. Acute pancreatitis is more common in adults than in children.
   E. True.

16.15 A. True.
   B. True. In neonates the blood–brain barrier is relatively permeable and unconjugated bilirubin can accumulate in the lipid-rich brain tissue causing kernicterus (bilirubin encephalopathy).
   C. False. The excess bilirubin is mainly conjugated in the Dubin–Johnson syndrome.
   D. True. This is a pre-hepatic cause of jaundice.
   E. True. These include Gilbert's syndrome, Crigler–Najjar syndrome, Dubin–Johnson syndrome and Rotor syndrome.

17

Endocrine system

17.1 Parathyroid adenomas:

    A. Are more common in women than in men.

    B. Are usually multiple.

    C. Produce calcitonin.

    D. Are most frequently situated in the superior glands.

    E. Cause resorption of bone tissue.

17.2 Cushing's syndrome:

    A. Is not associated with signs of virilism.

    B. May be due to an adrenal cortical adenoma.

    C. May be associated with oat-cell carcinoma of the lung.

    D. Causes decreased breakdown of body protein.

    E. Is characterised by raised levels of cortisol.

17.3 Hashimoto's disease of the thyroid:

    A. Shows a massive lymphoid infiltrate when examined microscopically.

    B. Is considered to be an autoimmune disease.

    C. Is not associated with autoimmune gastritis.

    D. Is associated with autoimmune adrenalitis (Addison's disease).

    E. May show Askanazy cells (Hurthle cells, oxyphil cells) when examined microscopically.

(Answers overleaf)

17.1 **A.** **True.** Parathyroid adenomas are three times as common in females as in males.
    B. **False.** Parathyroid adenomas are usually solitary lesions.
    C. **False.** The C-cells of the thyroid produce calcitonin. Functioning parathyroid adenomas elaborate parathormone.
    D. **False.** Some 75% of parathyroid adenomas arise in one of the inferior glands, 15% arise in the superior glands and the rest in anomalous positions such as the mediastinum.
    E. **True.** Parathormone causes an increase in osteoclastic activity leading to resorption of bone.

17.2 **A.** **False.** Cushing's syndrome in females is usually accompanied by some signs of virilism such as masculine distribution of hair, acne, deepening of the voice and oligomenorrhoea.
    B. **True.** A cortical adenoma may secrete cortisol and may escape the usual feedback mechanisms of control. Cortical adenomas account for about 5% of cases of Cushing's syndrome.
    C. **True.** Oat-cell carcinoma of the lung may produce an ACTH-like substance which stimulates the adrenals to produce too much cortisol. Other tumours which may do this include carcinoids, thymic and pancreatic tumours.
    D. **False.** There is increased catabolism of body protein leading to thinning of the skin, osteoporosis and muscular weakness.
    E. **True.** This is the essential biochemical finding in Cushing's syndrome.

17.3 **A.** **True.** This is the characteristic histological appearance of Hashimoto's disease.
    B. **True.** Auto-antibodies against thyroglobulin and a membrane component of the endoplasmic reticulum of thyroid epithelial cells are found in most cases of Hashimoto's thyroiditis.
    C. **False.** Hashimoto's thyroiditis is associated with autoimmune gastritis.
    D. **True.** In both of these conditions there is evidence of cell-mediated autoimmunity to mitochondrial antigens which are not entirely organ-specific.
    E. **True.** These cells are a characteristic feature of Hashimoto's thyroiditis.

17.4 Type I diabetes mellitus:
A. Tends to occur at an older age than does type II diabetes.
B. Is associated with increased production of glucagon.
C. Is usually treated with oral hypoglycaemic agents.
D. May be complicated by a retinopathy.
E. Is caused by destruction of alpha cells in the pancreatic islets.

17.5 Addison's disease:
A. In the last century was commonly due to tuberculosis.
B. May result in hypovolaemia and hypotension.
C. If primary, is associated with reduced levels of adrenocorticotrophic hormone (ACTH).
D. Results in hypernatraemia.
E. Is associated with hypopigmentation of the skin.

(Answers overleaf)

17.4 **A.** **False.** Type I (insulin-dependent) diabetes used to be known as juvenile-onset diabetes and it tends to occur at an earlier age than type II (non-insulin-dependent, maturity-onset) diabetes.

B. **False.** Diabetes mellitus is associated with a decrease in insulin production and a subsequent hyperglycaemia. Glucagon production will also be decreased.

C. **False.** Type I diabetes requires insulin therapy in the vast majority of cases.

D. **True.** The microangiopathy associated with diabetes mellitus may produce considerable damage to the retina.

E. **False.** Diabetes mellitus is caused by destruction of beta cells in the islets of Langerhans in the pancreas.

17.5 **A.** **True.** When Addison first described the disease (in 1855) tuberculous destruction of the adrenals was the commonest cause. Today autoimmunity is the commonest cause.

B. **True.** Mineralocorticoid deficiency results in loss of salt and water with consequent hypovolaemia and hypotension.

C. **False.** In primary hypoadrenalism the adrenals are the failing part of the system, and ACTH levels will be raised in an attempt to get the adrenals to produce more steroid hormones.

D. **False.** *Hypo*natraemia is a feature of Addison's disease due to failure of reabsorption of salt in the renal tubules.

E. **False.** *Hyper*pigmentation of the skin occurs in Addison's disease, particularly on the external genitalia and exposed areas of skin.

17.6 **Primary hyperparathyroidism:**
  A. Is usually due to a parathyroid adenoma.
  B. Features reduced levels of parathormone.
  C. Is associated with duodenal ulceration.
  D. Often presents with symptoms relating to renal stones.
  E. May cause tetany.

17.7 **In the pituitary gland:**
  A. Somatotroph cells produce growth hormone.
  B. Functional adenomas are most commonly composed of corticotroph cells.
  C. Non-functional adenomas are the commonest cause of hypopituitarism.
  D. Growth-hormone-producing adenomas cause acromegaly if they occur before puberty.
  E. Post-partum haemorrhage may cause pituitary necrosis.

17.8 **The following are recognised complications of diabetes mellitus:**
  A. Amyloid deposition.
  B. Glomerulosclerosis.
  C. Peripheral vascular disease.
  D. Pyelonephritis.
  E. Blindness.

(Answers overleaf)

17.6 **A.** **True.** A parathyroid adenoma is the commonest cause of primary hyperparathyroidism. Other causes include hyperplasia of the parathyroid glands or occasionally parathyroid carcinoma.

B. **False.** Levels of parathormone are raised in primary hyperparathyroidism.

C. **True.** Duodenal ulceration occurs in about 15% of subjects with hyperparathyroidism. This is thought to be due to the enhancing effect which hypercalcaemia has on the hormone gastrin.

D. **True.** About half the subjects with primary hyperparathyroidism present with symptoms relating to renal stones.

E. **False.** Tetany occurs with hypocalcaemia such as may occur in hypoparathyroidism.

17.7 **A.** **True.** These cells, which are acidophilic on conventional staining, stain strongly for growth hormone using immunocytochemical techniques.

B. **False.** Prolactinomas are the commonest type of functional adenoma. They account for about 60% of all pituitary adenomas.

C. **True.** The two other relatively common causes of hypopituitarism are Sheehan's syndrome and the empty sella syndrome.

D. **False.** Growth-hormone-producing adenomas cause gigantism if they occur before puberty and acromegaly after puberty.

E. **True.** This is called Sheehan's syndrome. Failure of lactation may be the presenting syndrome.

17.8 **A.** **False.** Amyloid deposition is not directly attributable to diabetes mellitus.

B. **True.** Glomerulosclerosis occurs secondarily to the microangiopathy in renal vasculature.

C. **True.** Peripheral vascular disease occurs because of the accelerated atheroma that occurs in diabetes and the microangiopathy.

D. **True.** Resistance to infections is decreased in subjects with diabetes mellitus and so pyelonephritis occurs with an increased frequency.

E. **True.** Blindness may result from the effect of the microangiopathy on the retinal vessels and visual acuity may be diminished by cataract formation.

17.9 Phaeochromocytomas:

A. Are derived from adrenocortical cells.
B. Are classified as paragangliomas.
C. Cause hypertension by excessive production of aldosterone.
D. May cause sweating and nervousness.
E. May be familial.

17.10 Graves' thyroiditis:

A. Usually occurs with a thyroid of normal size.
B. Is caused by an excess of thyroid-stimulating hormone (TSH).
C. Has a positive association with pretibial myxoedema.
D. Has a histological picture of hypoplastic acinar epithelium.
E. Has a positive association with exophthalmos.

17.11 Papillary carcinoma of the thyroid:

A. Occurs most frequently in the elderly.
B. Is the least common type of thyroid carcinoma.
C. Has a prognosis worse than that of follicular thyroid carcinoma.
D. May contain psammoma bodies.
E. Metastasises most commonly by the haematogenous route.

(Answers overleaf)

17.9 **A.** **False.** Phaeochromocytomas are derived from the cells of the adrenal medulla.

B. **True.** Other abdominal paragangliomas include those arising from the organs of Zuckerkandl.

C. **False.** Phaeochromocytomas may cause hypertension but do so by excessive production of catecholamines. Conn's syndrome is hypertension caused by excessive production of aldosterone.

D. **True.** These symptoms may be attributed to excessive production of catecholamines.

E. **True.** Phaeochromocytomas may be part of the multiple endocrine neoplasia (MEN) syndrome.

17.10 **A.** **False.** Graves' disease usually produces a diffuse goitre.

B. **False.** Graves' disease is caused by an auto-antibody which binds to thyroid epithelial cells and mimics the action of TSH.

C. **True.** This name is rather misleading since it occurs in this form of hyperthyroidism rather than in hypothyroidism. The appearance is due to an accumulation of mucopolysaccharides in the dermis.

D. **False.** The acinar epithelium will be hyperplastic due to the stimulatory effect of the auto-antibody.

E. **True.**

17.11 **A.** **False.** Papillary carcinoma of the thyroid usually occurs before the age of 45 years.

B. **False.** Papillary carcinoma is the most common malignant tumour of the thyroid.

C. **False.** Papillary carcinoma has, on average, a better prognosis than its follicular counterpart.

D. **True.** Psammoma bodies are concentrically-lamellated calcific bodies which are found in papillary tumours of the thyroid, ovary and meninges.

E. **False.** Papillary carcinoma rarely metastasises by the blood; lymphatic metastasis to cervical lymph nodes may occur but can still be associated with a good prognosis.

17.12 Hypoparathyroidism:
  A. Occurs in the di George syndrome.
  B. Is accompanied by decreased plasma phosphate levels.
  C. May occur after thyroidectomy.
  D. May produce tetany.
  E. May be due to organ-specific autoimmunity.

17.13 Insulin:
  A. Promotes glycogen breakdown in the liver.
  B. Promotes glucose entry into cells.
  C. Is produced by the alpha cells in the islets of Langerhans.
  D. Promotes lipolysis.
  E. Promotes gluconeogenesis.

17.14 The following are recognised complications of diabetes mellitus:
  A. Kimmelstiel–Wilson lesions in the kidneys.
  B. Retinopathy.
  C. Pre-eclamptic toxaemia.
  D. Accelerated atheroma.
  E. Peripheral neuropathy.

(Answers overleaf)

17.12 A. True. In the di George syndrome there is congenital absence of the parathyroid glands.
B. False. Plasma phosphate levels are increased.
C. True. Damage or removal of the parathyroid glands may occur during thyroidectomy.
D. True. Spasm of skeletal muscles may occur in the hypocalcaemic state that accompanies hypoparathyroidism.
E. True. Idiopathic hypoparathyroidism is thought to be due to destruction of the glands by an auto-antibody.

17.13 A. False. Insulin promotes glycogen synthesis. Glucagon promotes glycogen breakdown in the liver.
B. True.
C. False. Insulin is produced by the beta cells in the islets of Langerhans, glucagon is produced by the alpha cells.
D. False. Insulin inhibits lipolysis and promotes lipogenesis.
E. False. Glucagon promotes gluconeogenesis.

17.14 A. True. This is the eponymous term for nodular glomerulosclerosis.
B. True. This is due to disease of small vessels in the retina.
C. True. Neonatal hypoglycaemia and large babies are other complications that may occur in babies of diabetic mothers.
D. True. This accounts for 80% of adult diabetic deaths from mechanisms such as myocardial infarction, cerebrovascular disease and limb ischaemia.
E. True. This may be due to occlusion of the small vessels supplying nerves.

18

Breast

18.1 Breast carcinoma:

A. Is less common in women who give birth before the age of 18 years compared with those who give birth after the age of 30 years.

B. Is most commonly found in the lower outer quadrant of the breast.

C. Has a better prognosis if of a tubular, rather than ductal, type.

D. Has a better prognosis if positive for oestrogen receptors.

E. May be associated with microcalcification.

18.2 The terminal ductal lobular unit:

A. Contains myoepithelial cells.

B. Contains lactiferous ducts.

C. Secretes glycoproteins in the non-pregnant state.

D. Is present in the male breast.

E. Produces milk.

18.3 The following changes in the breast are associated with an increased risk of developing breast cancer:

A. Atypical epithelial hyperplasia.

B. Apocrine metaplasia.

C. Sclerosing adenosis.

D. Fibrosis.

E. Florid epithelial hyperplasia without atypia.

(Answers overleaf)

18.1 **A.** **True.**   The risk for those who give birth before 18 years is one-third that of those who give birth after the age of 30 years.

B. **False.**   The most common site is the upper outer quadrant (50% of tumours). Only about 10% of breast carcinomas occur in the lower outer quadrant.

C. **True.**   Tubular carcinoma has a significantly more favourable prognosis than the more common ductal type.

D. **True.**   Oestrogen receptor positivity is associated with a better prognosis, probably because it is most common in well-differentiated tumours.

E. **True.**   This microcalcification is the main justification for mammographic screening.

18.2 **A.** **True.**   These cells are contractile and are involved in the mechanical expression of milk.

B. **False.**   The lactiferous ducts are large ducts which converge upon the nipple; there are 15–20 of them in each breast.

C. **True.**   The epithelial cells in the terminal ductal lobular unit are producing glycoproteins all the time.

D. **False.**   The male breast contains only ductal structures and has a similar appearance to the prepubertal female breast.

E. **True.**   This is the main function of the breast, and the milk is produced by the epithelial cells lining the acini in the terminal ductal lobular unit.

18.3 **A.** **True.**   Atypical epithelial hyperplasia is recognised to be associated with a five times greater risk of developing breast cancer.

B. **False.**   Apocrine metaplasia ('pink cell change') has not been shown to be associated with an increased risk of developing breast cancer.

C. **False.**   The importance of sclerosing adenosis lies in its ability to cause a clinical breast lump and to have some resemblance to carcinoma in histological sections, particularly sections performed using rapid freezing methods.

D. **False.**   Fibrosis does not have a proven association with increased risk of developing breast carcinoma.

E. **True.**   There is an increased risk of developing breast cancer in subjects with florid epithelial hyperplasia without atypia, which is about twice that of the general population.

18.4 **In the UK breast cancer screening programme:**
  A. All women over 50 years of age are invited to attend.
  B. Participants are screened every 2 years.
  C. Mammography is the screening modality.
  D. Histopathologists are not a necessary part of the service.
  E. Screen-detected carcinomas should, on average, be smaller than non-screen-detected lesions.

18.5 **Fat necrosis in the breast:**
  A. Occurs more frequently in pre-menopausal women than in post-menopausal women.
  B. Is commoner in thin, rather than obese, women.
  C. May clinically mimic carcinoma.
  D. Is thought to be caused by trauma.
  E. May lead to calcification.

18.6 **Fibroadenomas:**
  A. Are rare tumours of the breast.
  B. Have a peak incidence in the third decade of life.
  C. Are usually multiple.
  D. May grow rapidly during pregnancy.
  E. May be diagnosed by fine-needle aspiration cytology.

(Answers overleaf)

18.4 **A.** **False.** Women between the ages of 50 and 64 years are invited to attend for screening.
  B. **False.** The screening occurs on a 3-yearly cycle.
  C. **True.** Microcalcification and soft tissue distortion are the mammographic abnormalities which are sought.
  D. **False.** Once a lesion has been detected on mammograms its nature must be established by clinical examination and histological diagnosis.
  E. **True.** This is the rationale behind breast screening.

18.5 **A.** **False.** Fat necrosis is more common in post-menopausal women.
  B. **False.** Fat necrosis is more common in obese women.
  C. **True.** Fat necrosis may present as a discrete immobile lump with ill-defined margins and so can mimic carcinoma.
  D. **True.** Trauma is thought to be the cause, with mechanical disruption of adipocytes, but a history of trauma is not always elicited.
  E. **True.** This may be seen on mammography.

18.6 **A.** **False.** Fibroadenomas are the commonest benign tumours of the breast.
  B. **True.**
  C. **False.** Fibroadenomas are usually solitary; there are uncommon instances of multiple lesions.
  D. **True.** Fibroadenomas are influenced by the hormonal milieu and so may grow fast during pregnancy, a feature which may mimic carcinoma.
  E. **True.** An adequate aspiration of a fibroadenoma has characteristic cytological appearances which allow a confident diagnosis to be made, after which the lesions may be left in situ.

18.7 Mammary duct ectasia:
  A. May cause nipple retraction.
  B. Is characterised histologically by acute inflammation without fibrosis.
  C. Is most frequent in women in the third decade of life.
  D. Has a positive association with nulliparity.
  E. May produce a blood-stained nipple discharge.

18.8 Gynaecomastia:
  A. Occurs most frequently in the third decade of life.
  B. Has histological appearances which include stromal oedema and epithelial proliferation.
  C. Is associated with endocrine disturbances.
  D. Has been associated with treated prostatic carcinoma.
  E. May occur with chlorpromazine administration.

18.9 Duct papillomas:
  A. Are the commonest cause of nipple discharge.
  B. Arise from lobular epithelium.
  C. When solitary, are not premalignant.
  D. Arise most frequently in the second decade of life.
  E. Are more common than fibroadenomas.

(Answers overleaf)

18.7   **A.**   **True.**   Fibrosis around the ectatic ducts may lead to nipple retraction.
     B.   **False.**   The inflammation is chronic with marked fibrosis.
     C.   **False.**   Duct ectasia occurs predominantly after the age of 30 years.
     D.   **False.**   Women with duct ectasia are usually parous.
     E.   **True.**   This sign is a mimic of intraduct carcinoma and careful histological examination is required to distinguish between the two.

18.8   **A.**   **False.**   Gynaecomastia occurs most frequently at puberty and in old age.
     B.   **True.**   These are the typical histological appearances, although hyalinised connective tissue may replace the stromal oedema in older lesions.
     C.   **True.**   Gynaecomastia is associated with hyperthyroidism, pituitary disorders, and adrenal or testicular tumours.
     D.   **True.**   Stilboestrol has been used to treat prostatic carcinoma and this may produce gynaecomastia.
     E.   **True.**

18.9   **A.**   **True.**   Some 80% of duct papillomas present with nipple discharge. Other causes of nipple discharge include duct ectasia and intraduct carcinoma.
     B.   **False.**   They arise from the epithelium lining large ducts, usually within 40 mm of the nipple.
     C.   **True.**   There is a rare variant with multiple peripheral duct papillomas which does carry an increased risk of carcinoma.
     D.   **False.**   Duct papillomas have a peak incidence in middle-aged women.
     E.   **False.**   Fibroadenomas are considerably more common than duct papillomas.

18.10 Intralobular carcinoma (lobular carcinoma in situ):
- **A.** Usually presents as a discrete lump.
- **B.** Occurs predominantly in post-menopausal women.
- **C.** Rarely progresses to invasive carcinoma.
- **D.** Is characterised histologically by distended acini without invasion.
- **E.** Has a comedo variant.

18.11 Paget's disease of the nipple:
- **A.** Presents clinically with eczema or erosion of the nipple.
- **B.** Is associated with underlying carcinoma.
- **C.** Occurs in about 20% of all breast carcinomas.
- **D.** Is characterised by malignant cells in the epidermis with pale cytoplasm.
- **E.** May affect the skeletal system.

18.12 Phyllodes tumours:
- **A.** Occur in a younger age group than fibroadenomas.
- **B.** Present as a discrete lump.
- **C.** Are distinguished from fibroadenomas by a less cellular stroma.
- **D.** Metastasise predominantly by the lymphatic route.
- **E.** Were previously known as giant fibroadenomas.

(Answers overleaf)

18.10 A. False. Unless an invasive tumour is also present then intralobular carcinoma rarely presents as a lump. It is often found incidentally in biopsies taken for other reasons, e.g. adjacent to benign lesions such as fibroadenomas.

B. False. Intralobular carcinoma is usually found in premenopausal women. If found in post-menopausal women there is usually an associated invasive component.

C. False. Roughly one-third of patients who have intralobular carcinoma treated by less than a mastectomy will go on to develop invasive carcinoma, and this risk is increased for the contralateral breast as well.

D. True. These are the characteristic histological appearances.

E. False. Necrosis is rare in intralobular carcinoma. The comedo variant occurs in intraduct carcinoma.

18.11 A. True. These are the usual clinical appearances.

B. True. This carcinoma may be of intraduct or invasive type.

C. False. Paget's disease of the nipple occurs in about 2% of breast carcinomas.

D. True. These cells may contain intracytoplasmic mucin which can be demonstrated by special histological stains.

E. False. Paget's disease of the bone is an unrelated condition (save that Paget described it).

18.12 A. False. Although phyllodes tumours can present at any age the median age is 45 years, so they tend to occur in an older age group when compared with fibroadenomas.

B. True. A lump is the usual presenting feature.

C. False. The stroma of a phyllodes tumour is more cellular than that of a fibroadenoma, an important distinguishing feature in the histological diagnosis. The stroma of a phyllodes tumour may also show cellular pleomorphism and increased numbers of mitotic figures.

D. False. If phyllodes tumours metastasise then they do so predominantly by the haematogenous route.

E. True. This was not a very suitable name since phyllodes tumours are not invariably large and they have a histological appearance different to that of fibroadenomas.

18.13 Radial scars:

A. Are detected more commonly in pre- than post-menopausal women.

B. May be detected radiographically.

C. Often contain invasive carcinoma.

D. When smaller than 10 mm are named complex sclerosing lesions.

E. Contain foci of epithelial proliferation.

(Answers overleaf)

18.13 A. False.   Radial scars are more commonly detected in post-rather than pre-menopausal women.

   B. True.   This is the usual way in which radial scars are detected so their detected incidence has increased with the introduction of the NHS Breast Screening Programme.

   C. False.   Radial scars are benign lesions which may radiographically mimic carcinoma.

   D. False.   If a radial scar is larger than 10 mm in maximum extent it is named a complex sclerosing lesion.

   E. True.   A radial scar is a stellate lesion with foci of epithelial cell proliferation.

19

Female genital tract

19.1 Cervical glandular intraepithelial neoplasia:

A. Is more common than squamous carcinoma in situ of the cervix.

B. May develop into invasive adenocarcinoma.

C. Has a positive association with use of the oral contraceptive pill.

D. Is more easily detected by cervical cytology than its squamous counterpart.

E. Is increasing in detected incidence.

19.2 Endometrial hyperplasia:

A. Is associated with obesity.

B. Of the simple type, is associated with an increased risk of endometrial adenocarcinoma.

C. Is associated with unopposed oestrogenic stimulation.

D. May be diagnosed clinically.

E. Is more common in post- than in pre-menopausal women.

19.3 Ovarian carcinoma:

A. Has an increased incidence in women who give birth before the age of 25 years.

B. Is the commonest fatal gynaecological malignancy.

C. Has a survival rate of over 50% at 5 years.

D. Which is aneuploid, has a better prognosis than diploid tumours.

E. Commonly spreads to the contralateral ovary.

(Answers overleaf)

19.1 **A.** **False.** Squamous neoplasia of the cervix is more common than glandular neoplasia.
  B. **True.**
  C. **True.**
  D. **False.** The glandular cells are further up the endocervical canal and may not be sampled by a cervical spatula.
  E. **True.** This may be a real increase in the incidence of the disease or may be due to increased recognition of glandular neoplasia.

19.2 **A.** **True.** Androstenedione is converted to oestrone by aromatase, which is an enzyme in fat cells, and the oestrone may stimulate endometrial hyperplasia.
  B. **False.** The complex atypical type of hyperplasia may progress to endometrial adenocarcinoma.
  C. **True.**
  D. **False.** Endometrial hyperplasia is a histological diagnosis made on the examination of endometrial curettings; it may only be suspected clinically.
  E. **False.** Endometrial hyperplasia occurs most commonly in pre- and peri-menopausal women.

19.3 **A.** **False.** Pregnancy before the age of 25 years is associated with a diminished risk of ovarian cancer.
  B. **True.** Although it is not the commonest gynaecological malignancy, ovarian carcinoma does account for the most deaths.
  C. **False.** The crude overall 5-year survival rate is about 35%.
  D. **False.** Aneuploid tumours pursue a more aggressive course than do their diploid counterparts.
  E. **True.** The peritoneal cavity and para-aortic lymph nodes are the other common sites of spread.

19.4 Cervical carcinoma:
- **A.** Is usually an adenocarcinoma.
- **B.** Is associated with infection by some types of human papillomavirus.
- **C.** May cause death due to uraemia.
- **D.** May arise from areas of cervical intraepithelial neoplasia.
- **E.** Rarely spreads to lymph nodes.

19.5 Endometrial carcinoma:
- **A.** Has an overall 5-year survival rate of about 36%.
- **B.** Has an increased incidence in women with oestrogenic ovarian tumours.
- **C.** Has a peak incidence in the sixth decade.
- **D.** Rarely invades the myometrium.
- **E.** Has a higher incidence in multiparous women.

19.6 The following statements about ovarian endometriosis are true:
- **A.** It is associated with multiparity.
- **B.** Ascites is the commonest presenting feature.
- **C.** It tends to regress after the menopause.
- **D.** It is characterised histologically by endometrial glands, endometrial stroma and haemorrhagic foci.
- **E.** It may be the site of origin of endometrioid-type carcinoma.

(Answers overleaf)

19.4 **A.** **False.** Some 95% of cervical carcinomas are squamous cell carcinomas.
B. **True.** Cervical carcinoma is associated with types 16 and 18 of the human papillomavirus. This may account for the epidemiology of the disease, which shows indicators of sexual promiscuity to be important risk factors.
C. **True.** Death may be caused by ureteric obstruction by tumour, leading to renal failure.
D. **True.** This is the rationale behind the programme of screening by cervical cytology.
E. **False.** Lymph node spread often occurs at a relatively early stage to the pelvic, inguinal and aortic lymph nodes. Blood-borne spread tends to occur at a later stage.

19.5 **A.** **True.** Individual prognosis is related to tumour differentiation and degree of spread (staging).
B. **True.** Oestrogen appears to be a contributory factor to the aetiology of endometrial carcinoma.
C. **True.** Endometrial carcinoma occurs most commonly between the ages of 50 and 60 years.
D. **False.** Endometrial carcinoma invades the myometrium at an early stage, but because the myometrium is thick the tumour is usually confined to the uterus until a late stage of the disease.
E. **False.** Endometrial carcinoma has a higher incidence in nulliparous women.

19.6 **A.** **False.** Ovarian endometriosis is associated with sterility and hence low parity.
B. **False.** Pain is the commonest presenting feature. Ascites is an infrequent complication.
C. **True.** Regression is usual after the menopause.
D. **True.** The presence of endometrial glands and stroma is necessary to make a definite histological diagnosis of endometriosis. In long-standing lesions only haemosiderin-laden macrophages may remain.
E. **True.** Carcinoma does, rarely, arise in deposits of endometriosis and the endometrioid type is the most frequent.

19.7 Complete hydatidiform mole:

A. Has a greater incidence in Europe when compared with Southeast Asia.

B. Is usually triploid on chromosomal analysis.

C. May progress to choriocarcinoma.

D. Always produces chorionic gonadotrophin.

E. May cause hyperthyroidism.

19.8 Uterine leiomyomas:

A. Are the commonest tumours of the female genital tract.

B. Are associated with high parity.

C. May cause subfertility.

D. May cause abnormal uterine bleeding.

E. May measure up to 200 mm in diameter.

19.9 The following tumours of the ovary are thought to be derived from germ cells:

A. Granulosa cell tumour.

B. Krukenberg tumour.

C. Brenner tumour.

D. Yolk sac tumour.

E. Endometrioid carcinoma.

(Answers overleaf)

19.7 **A.** **False.** The incidence in Europe is about 1 in 1000 deliveries but in Southeast Asia it may be as high as 1 in 100 deliveries.

B. **False.** Complete hydatidiform mole is diploid on chromosomal analysis. Partial hydatidiform mole is triploid.

C. **True.** Approximately 2% of subjects with complete hydatidiform mole will go on to develop choriocarcinoma.

D. **True.** Chorionic gonadotrophin, usually measured as the beta subunit of hCG, is very useful in determining the management of this condition.

E. **True.** Hyperthyroidism occasionally occurs due to a thyroid stimulator secreted by the hydatidiform mole. This stimulator may be part of the human chorionic gonadotrophin molecule.

19.8 **A.** **True.**

B. **False.** They are associated with low parity.

C. **True.** Submucosal leiomyomas may distort the uterine cavity and interfere with embryo implantation.

D. **True.** This is also due to distortion of the uterine cavity.

E. **True.** Leiomyomas are usually multiple and may vary in size from 5 to 200 mm or more in diameter.

19.9 **A.** **False.** Granulosa cell tumours are of the sex cord-stromal type.

B. **False.** Krukenberg tumours are metastatic deposits of adenocarcinoma (usually of gastric or colonic origin) with a surrounding desmoplastic reaction.

C. **False.** Brenner tumours are thought to be derived from the surface epithelium of the ovary.

D. **True.** Yolk sac tumours are thought to be derived from germ cells.

E. **False.** Endometrioid carcinomas are derived from the surface epithelium of the ovary.

19.10 The following ovarian tumours are malignant:

  A. Fibromas.
  B. Mature cystic teratomas.
  C. Brenner tumours.
  D. Krukenberg tumours.
  E. Mucinous cystadenocarcinomas.

19.11 Mucinous neoplasms of the ovary:

  A. May be lined by intestinal-type epithelium.
  B. Are usually unilocular.
  C. Occur more frequently than serous neoplasms of the ovary.
  D. May give rise to pseudomyxoma peritonei.
  E. Are bilateral in 50% of cases.

19.12 Ectopic pregnancy:

  A. Occurs most commonly in the ovary.
  B. May lead to a haemoperitoneum.
  C. May produce Arias-Stella changes in the endometrium.
  D. Is associated with chronic salpingitis.
  E. Can proceed to term.

(Answers overleaf)

19.10 A. False.   Fibromas are benign tumours arising from non-specialised fibrous tissue in the ovary.
   B. False.   Mature cystic teratomas ('dermoid cysts') are benign tumours. Rarely, malignant change may occur in a part of a mature teratoma (usually the squamous component).
   C. False.   Brenner tumours are benign tumours of transitional epithelium set in a fibrous stroma.
   D. True.   Krukenberg tumours are composed of metastatic carcinoma.
   E. True.   Cystadenocarcinomas are malignant epithelial tumours.

19.11 A. True.   Intestinal-type epithelium with goblet, Paneth and endocrine cells may be present.
   B. False.   Mucinous neoplasms are most commonly multilocular.
   C. False.   Serous neoplasms of the ovary are more common than the mucinous type.
   D. True.   Peritoneal seedlings from a mucinous cystadenocarcinoma may fill the peritoneal cavity with mucinous material and lead to intestinal obstruction.
   E. False.   Mucinous neoplasms of the ovary are bilateral in 10–20% of cases.

19.12 A. False.   The fallopian tube is the commonest site of ectopic pregnancy.
   B. True.   Rupture of an ectopic pregnancy can lead to haemorrhage into the peritoneal cavity.
   C. True.   If this change is seen in the endometrium without chorionic villi or fetal parts then the possibility of ectopic pregnancy should be considered.
   D. True.   Chronic salpingitis can lead to scarring of the fallopian tubes with disordered motility.
   E. True.   It is more usual for rupture to occur during the first trimester.

19.13 Gestational choriocarcinoma:

A. Is usually treated with radiotherapy.

B. Contains hydropic chorionic villi.

C. Often metastasises to the lungs.

D. Occurs after a complete hydatidiform mole in 50% of cases.

E. Usually spreads by lymphatic pathways.

(Answers overleaf)

19.13 A. False. Chemotherapy is the most common treatment modality and can achieve a high remission rate.

B. False. Choriocarcinoma is only composed of cytotrophoblast and syncytiotrophoblast; no chorionic villi are present.

C. True. Approximately 50% of gestational choriocarcinomas will have metastasised to the lungs at the time of presentation.

D. True. Some 25% arise after an abortion and the rest after previous ordinary pregnancies.

E. False. Haematogenous dissemination is the commonest route of spread.

20

Male genital tract

20.1 Lymphoma of the testis:
   A. Usually occurs below the age of 40 years.
   B. May produce bilateral testicular tumours.
   C. Accounts for over 50% of malignant testicular tumours.
   D. Histologically shows malignant cells predominantly within seminiferous tubules.
   E. Has a characteristic mottled macroscopic appearance.

20.2 Carcinoma of the penis:
   A. Is usually of squamous cell type.
   B. Is more common amongst Jewish than Moslem populations.
   C. May arise in areas of erythroplasia of Queyrat.
   D. Metastasises to inguinal lymph nodes.
   E. Has a peak incidence in the fourth decade of life.

20.3 Prostatic carcinoma:
   A. Is usually a squamous cell carcinoma.
   B. Often metastasises to the lumbar and sacral spine.
   C. Usually produces osteolytic bony metastases.
   D. Often shows regression with oestrogen therapy.
   E. Secretes alkaline phosphatase.

(Answers overleaf)

20.1 **A.** **False.** Testicular lymphomas usually occur over the age of 40 years and are the most common malignant testicular tumours in elderly males.

B. **True.** Lymphoma is the tumour type in 50% of subjects with bilateral testicular tumours.

C. **False.** Testicular lymphomas account for about 5% of all malignant testicular tumours.

D. **False.** Although some lymphoma cells may be found in tubules the malignant infiltrate is mainly interstitial.

E. **False.** Malignant lymphoma of the testis usually has a homogeneous macroscopic appearance.

20.2 **A.** **True.** Virtually all carcinomas of the penis are of squamous cell type.

B. **False.** In Jewish populations, where circumcision is usual in the first days of life, the incidence of carcinoma of the penis is lower than it is in Moslem populations, where circumcision is usual before the age of 10 years. Both of these populations have a much lower incidence of carcinoma of the penis than populations where circumcision is unusual.

C. **True.** Erythroplasia of Queyrat and Bowen's disease are both precursors of invasive carcinoma.

D. **True.** These nodes are the first site of lymphatic metastases.

E. **False.** Carcinoma of the penis usually affects men over the age of 40 years.

20.3 **A.** **False.** The overwhelming majority of prostatic carcinomas are of adenocarcinomatous type.

B. **True.** Prostatic carcinoma often metastasises to these bones by the retrograde venous route.

C. **False.** Bony metastases of prostatic carcinoma are usually sclerotic.

D. **True.** About 80% of prostatic cancers show regression of tumour growth with oestrogen therapy but later escape from this form of control.

E. **False.** Prostatic carcinoma usually secretes acid phosphatase which may be measured in the blood. Alkaline phosphatase may also be elevated but this is due to the non-specific effect of bony metastases.

20.4 Seminomas of the testes:
   A. Are common before puberty.
   B. Have an increased incidence in undescended testes.
   C. May contain teratomatous elements.
   D. Are usually very responsive to radiotherapy.
   E. Often metastasise to the inguinal lymph nodes.

20.5 Benign nodular hyperplasia of the prostate:
   A. Affects about three-quarters of men aged 70–80 years.
   B. Is characterised by glandular hypoplasia.
   C. Predisposes to the development of prostatic carcinoma.
   D. May cause renal failure.
   E. May contain areas of squamous metaplasia.

20.6 Idiopathic gangrene of the scrotum (Fournier's syndrome):
   A. Has a positive association with diabetes mellitus.
   B. Has a positive association with anal fistulae and ischiorectal abscesses.
   C. Usually affects young men.
   D. Is caused by group B streptococci.
   E. May involve the abdominal wall.

(Answers overleaf)

20.4 **A. False.** Seminoma of the testis very rarely occurs before puberty. It has a peak incidence between 30 and 50 years of age.

B. True. About 5% of testicular tumours arise in undescended testes.

C. True. Combined seminomas/teratomas account for about 15% of testicular tumours.

D. True. Seminomas are very radiosensitive. If spread has reached only the para-aortic lymph nodes then a cure rate of about 90% can be achieved by orchidectomy and radiotherapy.

E. False. The para-aortic lymph nodes are the usual site of lymphatic spread, following the testicular blood supply.

20.5 **A. True.** Benign nodular hyperplasia is a very common condition of the prostate in elderly men.

B. False. It is characterised by glandular *hyper*plasia together with stromal hyperplasia.

C. False. Benign nodular hyperplasia of the prostate is not a premalignant condition but prostatic carcinoma is quite common in the same age group.

D. True. Outflow obstruction of the bladder may lead to hydronephrotic kidneys with episodes of pyelonephritis leading to renal failure.

E. True. These areas of squamous metaplasia often surround areas of infarction.

20.6 **A. True.**

B. True.

C. False. It usually affects middle-aged and elderly men.

D. False. Faecal organisms are the causative agents, usually in a mixed infection with coliforms and *Bacteroides*.

E. True. The disease may spread to the abdominal wall, perineum and penis. When extensive it is often fatal.

20.7   Lymphogranuloma venereum:

    A. Is commoner in Europe than in the tropics.

    B. Is caused by *Treponema pallidum*.

    C. Often causes an inguinal lymphadenitis.

    D. Is diagnosed by dark-background microscopy of aspirated material.

    E. Causes condylomata acuminata.

20.8   Yolk sac tumour of the testes:

    A. Usually occurs in the second decade of life. < 3yrs

    B. Contains Schiller–Duval bodies.

    C. Contains α-fetoprotein.

    D. Is also known as orchioblastoma.

    E. May be a component of mixed germ-cell tumours.

(Answers overleaf)

20.7 **A.** **False.** Lymphogranuloma venereum is much commoner in the tropics than in Europe. Most cases seen in Britain have been acquired abroad.

B. **False.** *Treponema pallidum* is the causative organism of syphilis. Lymphogranuloma venereum is caused by *Chlamydia trachomatis* serotypes L1–L3.

C. **True.** Inguinal lymphadenitis is the usual manifestation of the disease 1–4 weeks after acquisition of the infection.

D. **False.** The spirochaetes which cause syphilis are seen by dark-background microscopy. Lymphogranuloma venereum may be diagnosed by Giemsa-stained smears of pus aspirated from the enlarged lymph nodes.

E. **False.** Condylomata acuminata are caused by subtypes of the human papillomavirus.

20.8 **A.** **False.** Pure yolk sac tumour of the testis usually occurs before the age of 3 years.

B. **True.** These are characteristic histological features composed of perivascular layers of tumour cells.

C. **True.** This may be demonstrated within tumour cells by immunohistochemistry or may be measured in the subject's serum prior to tumour excision.

D. **True.**

E. **True.**

21

Kidneys and urinary tract

21.1 The following factors predispose to pyelonephritis:
- **A.** Diabetes mellitus.
- **B.** Pregnancy.
- **C.** Vesico-ureteric reflux.
- **D.** Males less than 40 years old.
- **E.** Cystoscopy.

21.2 Alport's disease:
- **A.** Is inherited in an autosomal recessive pattern.
- **B.** Causes renal failure in females at an earlier age than in males.
- **C.** Produces deafness for high-frequency sounds.
- **D.** Has a positive association with corneal dystrophy.
- **E.** Results from defective tubular reabsorption of amino acids.

21.3 Renal carcinoma:
- **A.** Rarely invades the renal vein.
- **B.** Is more frequent in children than in adults.
- **C.** Is often composed of large cells with abundant clear cytoplasm.
- **D.** May present with haematuria.
- **E.** Is one of the tumours which often metastasises to bone.

(Answers overleaf) **167**

21.1 **A.** **True.** There is a general increased susceptibility to infection in subjects with diabetes mellitus, and glucose-containing urine is a good medium for bacterial growth.

B. **True.** There is a generalised relaxation of smooth muscle during pregnancy which may lead to reflux of urine up the ureters and so cause a pyelonephritis.

C. **True.** This is a potent predisposing factor for pyelonephritis.

D. **False.** From puberty to middle age there is a higher incidence of pyelonephritis amongst females compared with males. This is usually attributed to the shorter female urethra and to pregnancy.

E. **True.** Any instrumentation of the lower urinary tract increases the risk of pyelonephritis.

21.2 **A.** **False.** Alport's disease is an autosomal dominant condition with variable expression.

B. **False.** Males with Alport's disease usually develop renal failure at an earlier age than females with the condition.

C. **True.**

D. **True.** In severe cases of Alport's disease there may be dislocation of the lens, cataracts and corneal dystrophy.

E. **False.** The cause of Alport's disease is unknown but it may be due to defective synthesis of basement membrane. Defective tubular reabsorption of amino acids occurs in cystinuria.

21.3 **A.** **False.** Renal carcinoma commonly grows into the tributaries of the renal veins and may extend into the inferior vena cava (indicating a worse prognosis).

B. **False.** Renal carcinoma is more common in adults than in children.

C. **True.** Renal carcinoma is sometimes known as clear-cell carcinoma (other synonyms include Gravitz's tumour and hypernephroma).

D. **True.** Haematuria may occur if the tumour invades and ulcerates the renal pelvis.

E. **True.** The other tumours which often metastasise to bone include breast, prostatic, thyroid and lung carcinomas.

21.4 Transitional cell carcinomas of the bladder:

A. Are increased in incidence amongst workers in the aniline dye industry.
B. Have a positive association with cigarette smoking.
C. Have an increased incidence in Egypt.
D. May present with haematuria.
E. Often have a papillary structure.

21.5 In minimal-change disease of the glomeruli:

A. The incidence is greatest between the ages of 2 and 4 years.
B. Fusion of the foot processes of podocytes is seen on electron microscopy.
C. A non-selective proteinuria is usual.
D. Light microscopy shows crescent formation in glomeruli.
E. Cells of the proximal tubules contain lipid droplets.

21.6 Urinary calculi:

A. May cause hydronephrosis.
B. Are more common in temperate than tropical climates.
C. May induce squamous metaplasia in surrounding urothelium.
D. Are most commonly made of uric acid.
E. Are rarely made of calcium oxalate compounds.

(Answers overleaf)

21.4 **A. True.**   2-Naphthylamine appears to be the incriminated substance. The incidence is also increased in workers in the rubber industry.
   B. True.   There is an increased incidence amongst cigarette smokers.
   C. False.   There is a high incidence of bladder tumours in Egypt (thought to be induced by chronic schistosomiasis) but these are squamous rather than transitional cell carcinomas.
   D. True.   This is often the presenting feature.
   E. True.   A papillary pattern is the most usual form of transitional cell carcinoma. Less well differentiated tumours may have a predominantly solid growth pattern.

21.5 **A. True.**   Minimal-change disease can occur at any age but it is most frequent in early childhood.
   B. True.   Light microscopy usually shows no glomerular abnormality, but fusion and loss of foot processes of the podocytes may be seen on electron microscopy.
   C. False.   A selective proteinuria, with relatively low molecular weight proteins such as albumin, is usual in minimal-change disease. Diseases which damage the glomeruli more severely produce a non-selective proteinuria with proteins of all molecular weights.
   D. False.   Light microscopy usually shows no glomerular abnormality. Crescent formation is a feature of rapidly progressive glomerulonephritis.
   E. True.   This appearance gives rise to the older syndrome of lipoid nephrosis.

21.6 **A. True.**   Obstruction of urinary outflow leads to dilatation of the renal pelvis.
   B. False.   Urinary calculi are more common in tropical than in temperate climates because deposition is favoured by a highly concentrated urine.
   C. True.   Squamous cell carcinoma may develop in these metaplastic areas.
   D. False.   Only about 6% of urinary calculi are composed of uric acid.
   E. False.   Most urinary calculi are made mainly of calcium oxalate, often mixed with calcium phosphate and uric acid.

21.7 In chronic glomerulonephritis:

A. The subcapsular surface of the kidney is often finely granular.
B. The calyces and renal pelvis are usually distorted.
C. The kidneys are often enlarged.
D. There is often no history of preceding renal disease.
E. Many glomeruli are hyalinised.

21.8 The nephrotic syndrome:

A. May be caused by renal amyloidosis.
B. Is usually associated with a protein loss of less than 5 g per day.
C. Is associated with hypolipidaemia.
D. In children, is usually due to minimal-change glomerulonephritis.
E. Is characterised by proteinuria, hypoalbuminaemia and oedema.

21.9 Wilms' tumour (nephroblastoma):

A. Involves both kidneys in about 5% of cases.
B. Usually presents as an abdominal mass.
C. Rarely metastasises to the lung.
D. Has a 2-year survival rate of about 90%.
E. Usually affects adults.

(Answers overleaf)

21.7 **A.** **True.** This is the characteristic macroscopic appearance in chronic glomerulonephritis.

B. **False.** The calyces and renal pelvis are not usually distorted and this provides a useful macroscopic distinction from chronic pyelonephritis.

C. **False.** The kidneys are usually shrunken due to diffuse thinning of the cortex.

D. **True.** In over 70% of patients with chronic glomerulonephritis there is no history of the preceding renal disease which has been progressing silently until all the functional reserve of the kidney has been depleted.

E. **True.** Many glomeruli will be completely hyalinised, the remaining glomeruli may be hypertrophied.

21.8 **A.** **True.** Deposition of amyloid around the glomerular capillary basement membrane renders it more permeable to protein.

B. **False.** In adults with the nephrotic syndrome the urinary loss is usually more than 10 g per day.

C. **False.** A common feature of the nephrotic syndrome is *hyper*lipidaemia.

D. **True.** Minimal-change glomerulonephritis is the commonest cause of the nephrotic syndrome in children. In adults, acute diffuse, membranous and minimal-change glomerulonephritis are about equally common causes.

E. **True.** These are the main features of the nephrotic syndrome.

21.9 **A.** **True.** This bilateral involvement may occur by direct spread or synchronous tumours arising in areas of persistent blastema.

B. **True.** Abdominal mass is the commonest presentation. Other presenting symptoms include fever and haematuria.

C. **False.** Wilms' tumour commonly invades blood vessels and metastasises to the lungs.

D. **True.** Treatment by nephrectomy, radiotherapy and chemotherapy can achieve an apparent cure even when pulmonary metastases are present.

E. **False.** Wilms' tumour is a predominantly childhood tumour. It is the third commonest solid organ tumour in children under the age of 10 years.

21.10 Bilateral renal agenesis (Potter's syndrome):

A. Is associated with polyhydramnios.
B. Is associated with pulmonary hypoplasia.
C. Often results in a stillborn infant.
D. Is caused by failure of development of the ureteric bud.
E. Produces facial dysmorphology with low-set ears and receding chin.

21.11 Adult polycystic renal disease:

A. Has an autosomal dominant pattern of inheritance.
B. May be unilateral.
C. Has a positive association with berry aneurysms of the circle of Willis.
D. Causes renal failure in the first year of life.
E. Has a positive association with hepatic fibrosis.

21.12 Wegener's granulomatosis:

A. Occurs more commonly in males than in females.
B. May respond to cyclophosphamide therapy.
C. Is a necrotising vasculitis.
D. Is associated with typhoid.
E. May affect the upper respiratory tract as well as the kidneys.

(Answers overleaf)

21.10 A. False. Potter's syndrome produces oligohydramnios (paucity of amniotic fluid) because there is no production of fetal urine.
B. True. Other associated abnormalities include spinal cord defects.
C. True. Potter's syndrome is incompatible with life independent of the mother, and the infant is often stillborn.
D. True.
E. True. These are the characteristic external features of Potter's syndrome.

21.11 A. True. Childhood polycystic disease has an autosomal recessive pattern of inheritance.
B. False. Adult polycystic renal disease always affects both kidneys.
C. True. Death from subarachnoid haemorrhage, due to rupture of one of these aneurysms, is quite common.
D. False. Renal failure occurs in later life in adult polycystic renal disease; the onset of renal failure in childhood polycystic disease is much earlier.
E. False. There are often cysts in the liver in adult polycystic disease but hepatic fibrosis is not a feature. Substantial hepatic fibrosis, compromising hepatic function, may occur in childhood polycystic disease.

21.12 A. True. Wegener's granulomatosis is more common in males than in females. The fourth and fifth decades are the most commonly affected age groups.
B. True. Cyclophosphamide therapy produces an improvement in most patients and may reverse the glomerular damage if it is started early enough.
C. True. This is the characteristic histological feature.
D. False. The cause of Wegener's granulomatosis is unknown. Adult haemolytic-uraemic syndrome may occur after typhoid infection.
E. True.

22

Lymph nodes, thymus and spleen

22.1 The germinal centre of a lymph node:

A. Contains mainly T-lymphocytes.
B. Contains dendritic reticulum cells.
C. Generates immunoglobulin-producing plasma cells.
D. Is characteristically enlarged in established infectious mononucleosis.
E. Contains the cords and sinuses.

22.2 The following conditions may predispose to rupture of the spleen:

A. Road traffic accidents.
B. Sickle cell anaemia in adults.
C. Infectious mononucleosis.
D. Myelofibrosis.
E. Malaria.

22.3 Hodgkin's disease:

A. Is characterised histologically by the presence of Reed–Sternberg cells.
B. May be classified using the Rappaport classification.
C. Of the lymphocyte-depleted type is associated with the most favourable prognosis.
D. May be staged using the Ann Arbor system.
E. Usually presents with painless lymphadenopathy.

(Answers overleaf)

22.1 **A.** **False.** The germinal centres contain mainly B-lymphocytes.
    B. **True.** These are antigen-presenting cells which help to initiate a B-cell response to antigens entering the lymph node.
    C. **True.** These plasma cells are seen within the medullary cords.
    D. **False.** There is characteristically an expansion of the paracortex in infectious mononucleosis (and many other viral infections).
    E. **False.** These are situated in the medullary part of a lymph node.

22.2 **A.** **True.** Blunt abdominal trauma can cause rupture of the spleen, and an exploratory laparotomy is often indicated in such cases. Delayed rupture may occur after liquefaction of a subcapsular haematoma.
    B. **False.** In sickle cell anaemia there are repeated infarcts of the spleen producing splenic atrophy ('autosplenectomy').
    C. **True.** Spontaneous rupture of the spleen is a rare complication of infectious mononucleosis.
    D. **True.** There is often massive splenomegaly in myelofibrosis which predisposes to rupture.
    E. **True.** Massive splenomegaly may occur in malaria.

22.3 **A.** **True.** Reed–Sternberg cells are large, binucleate and have single large eosinophilic nuclear inclusions. They are essential for the diagnosis of Hodgkin's disease but similar cells may be found in other diseases.
    B. **False.** The Rappaport classification has been used to classify non-Hodgkin's lymphoma. The Rye and World Health Organization classifications are currently used to classify Hodgkin's disease.
    C. **False.** The lymphocyte-depleted type of Hodgkin's disease is associated with the worst prognosis.
    D. **True.** The Ann Arbor system divides Hodgkin's disease into four stages, according to its extent, with A or B subtypes according to the absence or presence of specified constitutional symptoms.
    E. **True.** Painless lymphadenopathy is the commonest presentation of Hodgkin's disease, usually in the cervical region.

22.4 Splenomegaly may occur in the following conditions:
   A. Gaucher's disease.
   B. Felty's syndrome.
   C. Amyloidosis.
   D. Hepatic cirrhosis.
   E. Niemann–Pick disease.

22.5 Congestive splenomegaly:
   A. May be caused by stenosis of the pulmonary valve.
   B. May be characterised histologically by Gamna–Gandy bodies.
   C. May be caused by hepatic cirrhosis.
   D. Occurs in pure left-sided heart failure.
   E. May be caused by thrombosis of the extrahepatic part of the portal vein.

22.6 Non-Hodgkin's lymphomas:
   A. Are derived mainly from B-lymphocytes.
   B. Usually present with painless lymphadenopathy.
   C. Usually present at an earlier age than does Hodgkin's disease.
   D. May be localised predominantly in the skin.
   E. May be classified using the Kiel classification.

(Answers overleaf)

22.4 A. True. In Gaucher's disease glucocerebrosides accumulate within phagocytic cells in the spleen to produce massive splenomegaly.

B. True. Splenomegaly and resultant hypersplenism may occur in Felty's syndrome.

C. True. Amyloid protein may accumulate in the spleen to produce a hard 'glassy' splenomegaly.

D. True. There is congestive splenomegaly in the portal hypertension which accompanies hepatic cirrhosis.

E. True. In Niemann–Pick disease lack of sphingomyelinase causes accumulation of sphingomyelin in the spleen.

22.5 A. True. Stenosis of the pulmonary valve may lead to right ventricular failure with a raised venous pressure transmitted back to the spleen causing a congestive splenomegaly.

B. True. These bodies represent healed infarcts and are composed of fibrous tissue with abundant haemosiderin deposition.

C. True. The portal hypertension which occurs in hepatic cirrhosis may cause a massive splenomegaly.

D. False. Pure left-sided heart failure will cause pulmonary oedema, but unless the right ventricle also fails there will not be raised systemic venous pressure.

E. True.

22.6 A. True. About 80% of non-Hodgkin's lymphomas appear to be derived from B-lymphocytes.

B. True. Painless lymphadenopathy is the commonest presentation.

C. False. The median age at presentation for non-Hodgkin's lymphoma is 50 years. Hodgkin's disease has a peak incidence in the second and third decades.

D. True. Mycosis fungoides and Sézary syndrome are examples of this.

E. True. The Kiel classification is the most recent of the many classifications that have been proposed for non-Hodgkin's lymphoma (others include the Rappaport and Lukes–Collin's classifications).

22.7 Burkitt's lymphoma:

A. Runs a prolonged course if untreated.
B. Rarely affects the jaw.
C. Is associated with infection by the Epstein–Barr virus.
D. Is a tumour of T-lymphocytes.
E. Has a geographical distribution which is very similar to that of falciparum malaria.

22.8 The following features may occur in Hodgkin's disease:

A. Pel–Ebstein fever.
B. Eosinophilia.
C. Askanazy cells.
D. Splenomegaly.
E. Pruritus.

22.9 In the di George syndrome:

A. The thymus is absent or a fibrous streak.
B. The parathyroids are present.
C. The abnormalities are caused by a failure of development of the epithelial components of the third and fourth pharyngeal pouches.
D. Cell-mediated immunity is normal.
E. There is a positive association with myasthenia gravis.

(Answers overleaf)

22.7 **A.** **False.** Untreated cases of Burkitt's lymphoma die quickly with widespread metastases to the liver, kidneys and other organs.
 B. **False.** The jaw is one of the commonest sites of Burkitt's lymphoma.
 C. **True.** It still has not been definitively proven that the Epstein–Barr virus (EBV) is the causative agent of Burkitt's lymphoma but serology and molecular biological evidence strongly suggest that it is.
 D. **False.** Burkitt's lymphoma is a tumour of B-lymphoblasts.
 E. **True.** Frequent attacks of malaria in childhood depress cellular immunity and it is thought that this may play a role in the development of Burkitt's lymphoma.

22.8 **A.** **True.** The Pel–Ebstein fever is characterised by a few days of high swinging pyrexia alternating with a few days when the patient is afebrile.
 B. **True.** Eosinophilia is a frequent finding in Hodgkin's disease.
 C. **False.** Askanazy cells occur in autoimmune thyroiditis. The characteristic cell in Hodgkin's disease is the Reed–Sternberg cell.
 D. **True.** Clinical splenomegaly occurs in about 50% of patients during the course of their disease.
 E. **True.** Pruritus is included as a constitutional symptom in the Ann Arbor staging classification. It occurs in about 25% of patients.

22.9 **A.** **True.**
 B. **False.** The parathyroids are absent. In Nezelof's syndrome the thymus is absent but the parathyroids are present.
 C. **True.** In Nezelof's syndrome there is failure of development of only the third pharyngeal pouch.
 D. **False.** There is greatly reduced cell-mediated immunity with marked vulnerability to infection.
 E. **False.** In myasthenia gravis there may be hyperplasia of the thymus or even a thymoma.

22.10 Extranodal lymphomas:

   A. Are most commonly sited in the gastrointestinal tract.

   B. Are mainly of T-cell differentiation.

   C. Often remain localised to a single organ for long periods of time.

   D. Which metastasise, often spread to sites of mucosa-associated lymphoid tissue.

   E. Are often Hodgkin's disease.

(Answers overleaf)

22.10 A. True. The gastrointestinal tract is the commonest site for extranodal lymphomas. They may occur anywhere else in the body but the other common sites are Waldeyer's ring, lungs, thyroid, salivary glands and skin.

B. False. They are mainly of B-cell differentiation. An important exception is the lymphoma associated with coeliac disease which is of T-cell differentiation.

C. True. For this reason extranodal lymphomas are often curable by surgery alone, which contrasts with the systemic nature of most nodal lymphomas.

D. True.

E. False. It is very rare for Hodgkin's disease to occur in an extranodal site.

23

Blood and bone marrow

23.1 Myelofibrosis:

A. Is characterised by increased numbers of fibroblasts in the bone marrow.
B. Is usually accompanied by splenic atrophy.
C. Often requires a trephine marrow biopsy for diagnosis.
D. Produces a low neutrophil alkaline phosphatase score.
E. Causes death most frequently by acute leukaemic transformation.

23.2 In haemophilia:

A. Purpura are a common finding. F   X linked recessive
B. The pattern of inheritance is autosomal recessive.
C. The blood clotting time is prolonged. T
D. Bleeding may be prevented by clotting factor replacement. T
E. In Britain there is a positive association with hepatitis C.

23.3 In hypoplastic (aplastic) anaemia:

A. The reticulocyte count is high in relation to the degree of anaemia.
B. Thrombocytopenia is present.
C. Blast cells are found in the peripheral blood.
D. The bone marrow is hypoplastic.
E. Of Fanconi type, inheritance is by a Mendelian dominant pattern.

23.1 **A.** **True.** The haemopoietic bone marrow is replaced largely by fibroblasts and a greatly increased amount of reticulin fibre.

B. **False.** Substantial splenomegaly is usually present due to extramedullary haemopoiesis.

C. **True.** Attempted aspiration of bone marrow often produces no material (a 'dry tap') and trephine biopsy is usually required to provide histological confirmation of the diagnosis.

D. **False.** The neutrophil alkaline phosphatase score is greatly elevated.

E. **False.** Some 10% of cases may transform into an acute leukaemia but death is more frequently due to myocardial infarction or some cerebrovascular catastrophe.

23.2 **A.** **False.** Purpura are not seen; they occur in bleeding disorders due to platelet dysfunction or deficiency.

B. **False.** Haemophilia (both types A and B) has a sex-linked recessive pattern of inheritance.

C. **True.** This is one of the characteristic laboratory findings.

D. **True.**

E. **True.** The frequent use of clotting factor replacements means that transmission of viral infections, such as hepatitis C or HIV, has been common.

23.3 **A.** **False.** The anaemia is due to lack of production of red blood cells, so the reticulocyte count is low in relation to the degree of anaemia.

B. **True.** Aplastic anaemia is characterised by a pancytopenia of which thrombocytopenia is a component.

C. **False.** No abnormal cells are found in the peripheral blood.

D. **True.** Trephine bone biopsy shows that over 75% of the marrow is composed of fat in aplastic anaemia.

E. **False.** Fanconi's anaemia follows a recessive pattern of inheritance.

23.4 Beta-thalassaemia major:
   A. Presents with anaemia at birth. F
   B. Produces a macrocytic anaemia. F
   C. Produces hepatosplenomegaly. T
   D. Rarely requires blood transfusion. F
   E. Is associated with extramedullary haemopoiesis. T

23.5 In acute leukaemias:
   A. Acute lymphoblastic leukaemia (ALL) occurs more frequently in adults than in children. F
   B. Anaemia is usually present. T
   C. Petechial haemorrhages are frequently present. thrombocytopenia
   D. The bone marrow is hypercellular. T Blast cells
   E. The meninges may provide a 'sanctuary' for leukaemic cells during chemotherapy.

23.6 Chronic lymphocytic leukaemia (CLL):
   A. Has a positive association with herpes zoster infections.
   B. Is associated with hypergammaglobulinaemia. hypo
   C. May produce Mikulicz's syndrome.
   D. Is characterised by a lymphopenia. F lymphocytosis
   E. May be complicated by a haemolytic anaemia.
              2y autoimmune haemolytic
                      anaemia in CLL

(Answers overleaf)

23.4 **A.** **False.** The anaemia appears at 3–6 months of age when there is the switch from production of fetal haemoglobin (with gamma chains) to adult haemoglobin (with beta chains).

B. **False.** A microcytic hypochromic anaemia is characteristic of beta-thalassaemia major.

C. **True.** Hepatosplenomegaly occurs due to extramedullary haemopoiesis and excessive red cell breakdown.

D. **False.** Beta-thalassaemia major requires regular blood transfusion to relieve the anaemia, and unless extensive chelation with desferrioxamine is used then iron overload ensues.

E. **True.** This may occur in the liver and spleen. Increased intramedullary haemopoiesis produces thinning of cortical bones and a characteristic facial appearance.

23.5 **A.** **False.** ALL is most frequent in children.

B. **True.** This anaemia may be manifest by pallor, weakness or fatigue.

C. **True.** A thrombocytopenia is usually present and petechial haemorrhages are common.

D. **True.** The hypercellular marrow is predominantly composed of blast cells.

E. **True.** Cranial (and in males testicular) irradiation may be required to eradicate leukaemic cells from these sites.

23.6 **A.** **True.** This is due to immune paresis.

B. **False.** There is reduction in the concentration of serum immunoglobulins (hypogammaglobulinaemia).

C. **True.** Infiltration of the lacrimal and salivary glands may produce this syndrome.

D. **False.** A lymphocytosis is the characteristic finding in the peripheral blood.

E. **True.** A secondary autoimmune haemolytic anaemia may develop.

23.7 Hereditary spherocytosis:

    A. Has a recessive pattern of inheritance.
    B. Has a positive association with cholesterol gallstones.
    C. Is characterised by a low reticulocyte count.
    D. Causes red cells to show decreased osmotic fragility.
    E. May be treated by splenectomy.

23.8 Vitamin B$_{12}$ deficiency:

    A. In Europe, is usually due to an autoimmune gastritis.
    B. Causes a megaloblastic anaemia.
    C. Has a positive association with Crohn's disease.
    D. May cause subacute combined degeneration of the spinal cord.
    E. May be caused by anti-convulsant drug therapy.

23.9 In pure iron deficiency:

    A. Macrocytes are commonly present in the blood film.
    B. The platelet count is usually reduced.
    C. Serum ferritin levels are raised.
    D. The total iron binding capacity (TIBC) is raised.
    E. Red blood cells are hypochromic.

(Answers overleaf)

23.7 **A.** **False.** Hereditary spherocytosis is inherited in an autosomal dominant pattern with variable penetration.

B. **False.** The incidence of pigment, rather than cholesterol, gallstones is increased in hereditary spherocytosis.

C. **False.** The reticulocyte count is raised to 5–20% because there is haemolysis of the spherocytes.

D. **False.** The osmotic fragility of the red blood cells is increased; this is an important diagnostic test.

E. **True.** Splenectomy usually produces a near-normal red blood cell life-span.

23.8 **A.** **True.** Pernicious anaemia (Addisonian anaemia) with an autoimmune gastritis is the commonest cause of vitamin B_{12} deficiency in Europe. In the Indian subcontinent veganism is an important factor.

B. **True.** There is a macrocytic anaemia with a hypercellular bone marrow in vitamin B_{12} deficiency.

C. **True.** Extensive ileal involvement by Crohn's disease may prevent absorption of vitamin B_{12}.

D. **True.** This neuropathy affects the peripheral sensory nerves and the posterior and lateral columns of the spinal cord.

E. **False.** Folate deficiency may be caused by drug therapy with anti-convulsants such as phenytoin.

23.9 **A.** **False.** Microcytic red blood cells are present in pure iron deficiency anaemia. Macrocytes are present only when there is a co-existent deficiency of folate or B_{12}.

B. **False.** There is usually some degree of thrombocythaemia in iron deficiency anaemia, particularly when chronic blood loss is the underlying cause.

C. **False.** Serum ferritin levels are low. Ferritin levels are raised in conditions of iron overload.

D. **True.** The saturation of the TIBC falls to less than 10%.

E. **True.** Target cells and poikilocytes may also be present.

23.10 Multiple myeloma:
- **A.** Usually produces sclerotic bony lesions.
- **B.** May produce proteinaceous casts in the renal tubules.
- **C.** Has a peak incidence in the fourth decade of life.
- **D.** Often produces Bence Jones proteinuria.
- **E.** May be complicated by systemic amyloidosis.

23.11 Chronic myeloid leukaemia (CML):
- **A.** Affects children more commonly than adults.
- **B.** Has a strong association with the Philadelphia chromosome.
- **C.** Is characterised by a high neutrophil alkaline phosphatase score.
- **D.** Has a median survival of less than a year.
- **E.** Usually produces a bone marrow with a hypocellular appearance.

23.12 Sickle cell anaemia:
- **A.** Is due to the substitution of valine for glutamine in position 6 of the beta chain of haemoglobin.
- **B.** Has a positive association with osteomyelitis.
- **C.** Is associated with splenomegaly in adults.
- **D.** May be complicated by aplastic crises.
- **E.** Provides some protection against *Plasmodium falciparum* malaria.

(Answers overleaf)

23.10 A. False. The bony lesions are lytic and appear as lucencies on radiographs.

B. True. These casts are surrounded by multinucleated giant cells and are a characteristic histological feature of 'myeloma kidney'.

C. False. The peak incidence is in the sixth decade with equal distribution between the sexes.

D. True. Immunoglobulin light chains are present in the urine of 60–80% of subjects with myeloma.

E. True. About 10% of cases develop systemic amyloidosis affecting the kidneys, tongue, heart and peripheral nerves.

23.11 A. False. The disease is most frequent between the ages of 50 and 60 years but it may occur in childhood.

B. True. The Philadelphia chromosome (translocation of the long arm of chromosome 22 to another chromosome, usually 9) is present in over 90% of subjects with chronic myeloid leukaemia.

C. False. The neutrophil alkaline phosphatase score is invariably low.

D. False. The median survival is 3–4 years. There is usually a transformation to an acute leukaemia.

E. False. The bone marrow is usually *hyper*cellular.

23.12 A. True. This is the molecular basis of the disease.

B. True. Osteomyelitis may develop in areas of infarcted bone.

C. False. Although the spleen may be enlarged in childhood, repeated infarcts produce splenic atrophy in adults ('autosplenectomy').

D. True. These aplastic crises occur after infection with parvoviruses or due to folate deficiency.

E. True. This may account for the geographical distribution of sickle cell anaemia.

23.13 **In glucose-6-phosphate dehydrogenase (G6PD) deficiency:**
   A. Haemolysis may be precipitated by primaquine.
   B. The deficiency is usually more severe in blacks than in Mediterraneans.
   C. The pattern of inheritance is sex-linked.
   D. Fava beans may precipitate haemolysis.
   E. Heinz bodies may be present.

23.14 **Vitamin K:**
   A. Occurs in high concentration in breast milk.
   B. Is found in green vegetables.
   C. Is essential for formation of clotting factors II, VII, IX and X.
   D. May not be absorbed in a subject with obstructive jaundice.
   E. Is synthesised by gut bacteria.

23.15 **Intravascular haemolytic transfusion reactions:**
   A. Occur with anti-A and anti-B antibodies.
   B. Occur with Rhesus antibodies.
   C. Require at least 500 ml of blood to be transfused before becoming evident.
   D. May cause oliguric renal failure.
   E. Should be treated with diuretics.

(Answers overleaf)

23.13 A. True. Primaquine, and other antimalarials such as quinine, may precipitate episodes of haemolysis.
B. False. The deficiency in blacks is often mild and is usually more severe in Mediterraneans.
C. True. G6PD deficiency affects males; female carriers have about half the normal red blood cell levels of G6PD.
D. True. Ingestion of fava beans produces an oxidant stress on the red blood cells, and the G6PD deficiency reduces the amount of reduced glutathione which opposes the oxidation.
E. True. These bodies are composed of oxidised denatured haemoglobin and may be seen in reticulocyte preparations.

23.14 A. False. Vitamin K is found only in low concentrations in breast milk and this, together with lack of bacteria in the neonatal gut, may lead to a vitamin K deficiency and haemorrhagic disease of the newborn.
B. True.
C. True. Without vitamin K these clotting factors are produced in an inactive form.
D. True. Subjects with obstructive jaundice require careful assessment of their blood coagulation before any invasive procedure to investigate or relieve their jaundice.
E. True.

23.15 A. True.
B. False. Rhesus antibodies, unlike anti-A and anti-B antibodies, are not complement fixing so intravascular haemolysis does not occur; red cells are taken up and destroyed in the reticulo-endothelial system.
C. False. Haemolytic transfusion reactions can occur with only a few millilitres of incompatible red cells.
D. True.
E. False. Intravenous fluids and steroids should be given after immediate cessation of transfusion.

24

Skin

24.1 Psoriasis:

A. Shows elongation of the rete ridges, Munro micro-abscesses and parakeratosis when examined microscopically.
B. Is sometimes associated with a polyarthritis.
C. Affects about 15% of the general population.
D. Is associated with pitting of the finger and toe nails.
E. Usually appears after 40 years of age.

24.2 Basal cell carcinoma of the skin:

A. Is sometimes known as 'rodent ulcer'.
B. Often metastasises.
C. Usually occurs in areas of skin that are not regularly exposed to the sun.
D. Histologically shows small dark cells with peripheral palisading.
E. May appear to have a multicentric origin.

24.3 Malignant melanoma:

A. Always contains melanin.
B. Rarely metastasises.
C. Usually occurs in childhood.
D. May occur as an 'in-situ' tumour.
E. Has a prognosis related to the depth of tumour invasion.

(Answers overleaf)

24.1 **A.** **True.** This is the typical histological picture. Munro micro-abscesses consist of accumulations of neutrophils in the parakeratotic horny layer.

B. **True.** About 5% of subjects with psoriasis develop a polyarthritis.

C. **False.** Psoriasis is estimated to affect about 2% of the general population.

D. **True.** About 25% of subjects with psoriasis have pitting of the finger and toe nails.

E. **False.** Psoriasis usually makes its first appearance between the ages of 15 and 30 years.

24.2 **A.** **True.** Basal cell carcinomas (BCCs) of the skin usually appear as ulcers with rolled margins.

B. **False.** Metastasis of a BCC is an exceedingly rare event.

C. **False.** BCCs usually occur on sun-exposed areas, especially on the face.

D. **True.** This is the characteristic histological appearance.

E. **True.** Some BCCs do appear to have a multicentric origin when examined histologically.

24.3 **A.** **False.** Some malignant melanomas contain no melanin (amelanotic melanomas).

B. **False.** Malignant melanoma has a great potential to metastasise by lymphatic and vascular routes.

C. **False.** Malignant melanoma is extremely rare before puberty.

D. **True.** Malignant melanocytes may be present at the dermoepidermal junction without invasion into the underlying dermis; an example is lentigo maligna or Hutchinson's melanotic freckle.

E. **True.** The depth of invasion may be assessed by measuring the thickest part of the tumour (Breslow's thickness) or by relating the depth of invasion to the surrounding skin appendages (Clark's levels).

24.4 **Squamous cell carcinoma of the skin:**

   A. Was a common tumour of early radiologists.
   B. Arises most commonly on the face, the back of the hands and the pinna of the ears.
   C. Is radiosensitive.
   D. Is associated with exposure to soot.
   E. May arise at the edges of long-standing ulcers.

24.5 **The following skin conditions are caused by viruses:**

   A. Impetigo.
   B. Molluscum contagiosum.
   C. Condylomata acuminata.
   D. Condylomata lata.
   E. Verruca vulgaris.

24.6 **The following dermatopathological definitions are correct:**

   A. Acanthosis — thickening of the epidermis.
   B. Hyperkeratosis — presence of nucleated squames in the horny layer.
   C. Pigment incontinence — loss of melanin from basal epidermal cells.
   D. Acantholysis — loss of cohesion between epidermal cells.
   E. Dyskeratosis — increase in thickness of the horny layer.

(Answers overleaf)

24.4 **A.** **True.** The first X-rays were of relatively low penetrance and caused squamous cell carcinomas on the skin of early radiologists who used their own bodies to calibrate their machines.
B. **True.** These are the commonest sites.
C. **True.** Surgical excision is the primary treatment of choice but radiotherapy provides an alternative.
D. **True.** Sir Percival Pott described squamous cell carcinomas of the scrotal skin in chimney sweeps.
E. **True.** These are called Marjolin's ulcers.

24.5 **A.** **False.** Impetigo is caused by group A β-haemolytic streptococci.
B. **True.** Molluscum contagiosum is caused by a poxvirus.
C. **True.** These condylomata are caused by some types of human papillomaviruses (HPV).
D. **False.** Condylomata lata occur in syphilis, the causative agent of which is *Treponema pallidum* (a spirochaete).
E. **True.** Verrucae are caused by HPVs of different types to those which cause condylomata acuminata.

24.6 **A.** **True.** Acanthosis describes an increase in thickness of the epidermis, due mainly to increase in thickness between the basal and granular layers.
B. **False.** Hyperkeratosis is an increase in the thickness of the horny layer. Parakeratosis describes the presence of nucleated squames in the horny layer.
C. **True.** The pigment from these cells may be ingested by macrophages in the upper part of the dermis.
D. **True.** This loss of cohesion may lead to the formation of vesicles and bullae.
E. **False.** Dyskeratosis is abnormal keratinisation of cells in the epidermis, usually below the level of the granular layer.

24.7 **Blue naevi:**
   A. Are usually multiple.
   B. Often undergo malignant transformation.
   C. Are composed of dendritic melanocytes.
   D. Are thought to arise from melanocytes arrested in their migration towards the epidermis.
   E. Feature a prominent epidermal component.

24.8 **Acne vulgaris:**
   A. Is an oestrogen-dependent disease.
   B. May be prevented by male castration.
   C. May be treated with retinoids.
   D. Affects the sweat glands of the axilla and groin.
   E. Often heals with scarring.

24.9 **Leprosy:**
   A. Is caused by *Mycobacterium bovis*.
   B. Affects about 10 million people in the world.
   C. Of the tuberculoid form, is more likely to be lethal than the lepromatous form.
   D. May produce autoamputations of digits.
   E. Of the tuberculoid form, is characterised histologically by a vigorous inflammatory response with granulomas.

(Answers overleaf)

24.7   **A.**   **False.**   Blue naevi are usually solitary.
        B.   **False.**   Malignant transformation is very rare.
        C.   **True.**   These dendritic melanocytes lie deep in the dermis and their heavy pigmentation leads to the blue appearance of the lesion.
        D.   **True.**   This is the most likely explanation of the origin of these naevi.
        E.   **False.**   An epidermal component is usually absent though sometimes a blue naevus can co-exist with a different type of naevus to produce a combined naevus.

24.8   **A.**   **False.**   Acne vulgaris is a testosterone-dependent disease, which is why it occurs more commonly in males than females.
        B.   **True.**   Eunuchs do not have acne but this approach to treatment is a little extreme.
        C.   **True.**   Synthetic analogues of retinoids, which modify keratin production, are effective at treating acne vulgaris. This suggests that keratin plugging of hair follicles may be the initial step in the disease process.
        D.   **False.**   Acne vulgaris affects the pilosebaceous units of the skin. Inflammation of the sweat glands occurs in the disease hidradenitis suppurativa.
        E.   **True.**   Although the active phase of acne vulgaris occurs in adolescence and young adulthood the scarring will persist.

24.9   **A.**   **False.**   Leprosy is caused by *Mycobacterium leprae*.
        B.   **True.**   Leprosy is still a considerable cause of morbidity on a world-wide scale but is rare in Britain where it occurs almost only as an imported disease.
        C.   **False.**   In the lepromatous form, the host immune response to the organism is deficient and death may occur from disseminated infection.
        D.   **True.**   This occurs due to the marked inflammatory response produced in the tuberculoid form of the disease.
        E.   **True.**

24.10 Lichen planus:

A. Is known to be an infectious disease.

B. May be treated with steroids.

C. Is characterised histologically by a band-like inflammatory cell infiltrate at the dermoepidermal junction.

D. Often affects the inner surface of the wrists.

E. May produce variable pigmentation of the skin.

(Answers overleaf)

24.10 A. False.   The cause of lichen planus is not known but no infectious agents have been identified.
  B. True.   Steroids usually induce regression of the disease.
  C. True.   This is the characteristic histological appearance.
  D. True.   This is a common site; mucosal surfaces may also be affected.
  E. True.   When the papules of lichen planus regress the skin may be left in a hyper- or hypopigmented state.

25

Osteoarticular and connective tissues

25.1 Acute osteomyelitis:

   A. Is most commonly caused by *Staphylococcus aureus*.
   B. Is not associated with subperiosteal abscesses.
   C. May be complicated by septicaemia.
   D. May result in the formation of sequestrum.
   E. Does not produce involucrum.

25.2 Osteosarcoma:

   A. Is rare in the metaphysis of long bones.
   B. Spreads most readily by the lymphatic pathways.
   C. May give a 'sunray spicule' appearance on radiographs.
   D. Is the commonest primary malignant bone tumour.
   E. Occurs most commonly between the ages of 10 and 25 years.

(Answers overleaf)

25.1 **A.** **True.** The staphylococcal strain responsible is often penicillin-resistant.

B. **False.** In children with osteomyelitis, pus from the medullary cavity may track through the cortex and then under the periosteum, which is only loosely attached to the underlying shaft during growth.

C. **True.** This is most likely to occur with staphylococcal osteomyelitis when production of coagulase may cause thrombosis in the vascular sinusoids in the marrow and lead to embolisation of this infected thrombus into the blood stream.

D. **True.** Accumulations of large amounts of pus under the periosteum may cause thrombosis of a nutrient artery with resultant ischaemic necrosis of the bone which may separate from the viable bone to form a sequestrum.

E. **False.** Involucrum is new bone formed beneath the periosteum which may be produced in the later stages of acute osteomyelitis.

25.2 **A.** **False.** The commonest site of osteosarcoma is in the metaphysis of long bones.

B. **False.** Lymph node metastases are unusual in osteosarcoma. The commonest pathway of spread is by the blood stream to the lungs.

C. **True.** Where the periosteum is raised, spicules of new bone are laid down at right angles to the bone shaft.

D. **True.**

E. **True.** Some 75% of cases fall within this age range.

25.3 Paget's disease of bone:

A. Rarely affects the skull.

B. May cause high-output cardiac failure.

C. May be complicated by the development of an osteosarcoma.

D. Is associated with lowered levels of serum alkaline phosphatase.

E. Usually appears before the age of 40 years.

25.4 Ankylosing spondylitis:

A. Is more common in females than in males.

B. Has a positive association with HLA-B27.

C. Usually affects elderly people.

D. May produce a uveitis.

E. Invariably produces a positive test for rheumatoid factor.

25.5 The features of osteoporosis include:

A. Decreased incidence of bony fractures.

B. An association with Cushing's syndrome.

C. A lack of active vitamin D.

D. Reduction in the mineralisation of bone.

E. Thinning of cortical bone.

(Answers overleaf)

25.3 **A.** **False.** The skull (together with the lumbar vertebrae, sacrum and pelvis) is one of the most commonly affected bones. An increase in head circumference, as evidenced by an increase in hat size, is a common finding.
  B. **True.** High-output cardiac failure may occur when Paget's disease is extensive and the blood flow through the affected bones and overlying skin is greatly increased.
  C. **True.** Paget's disease of bone is associated with a 30-fold increase in the risk of developing a sarcoma. The most common sarcoma is an osteosarcoma and the prognosis is usually poor with early metastasis to the lungs.
  D. **False.** Serum alkaline phosphatase activity is raised, indicating increased osteoblastic activity. Urinary hydroxyproline (an indicator of collagen breakdown) is increased in parallel with the alkaline phosphatase.
  E. **False.** Paget's disease of bone usually affects people over the age of 40 years.

25.4 **A.** **False.** Males are affected twice as frequently as females.
  B. **True.** Most subjects with ankylosing spondylitis have HLA-B27; this is the disease with one of the strongest associations with a particular HLA type.
  C. **False.** It usually affects young people.
  D. **True.** Back pain and an arthritis are the other prominent features.
  E. **False.** The serological findings are variable.

25.5 **A.** **False.** The incidence of fractures is increased. It is estimated that osteoporosis is a major factor in one million fractures every year in America.
  B. **True.** Osteoporosis occurs in Cushing's syndrome.
  C. **False.** A lack of vitamin D leads to osteomalacia rather than osteoporosis.
  D. **False.** The degree of mineralisation of bone in osteoporosis is normal but the total bone mass is reduced. Reduction in the mineralisation of bone occurs in osteomalacia.
  E. **True.** The radiographic appearance of osteoporosis may be similar to that seen in osteomalacia.

25.6 **In subjects with osteogenesis imperfecta:**
- **A.** There is abnormal synthesis of type I collagen.
- **B.** The sclerae may appear blue.
- **C.** Multiple fractures may occur in utero.
- **D.** The pattern of inheritance is always autosomal dominant.
- **E.** There is an increased incidence of hearing loss.

25.7 **Chondrosarcoma:**
- **A.** Is a malignant tumour showing osseous differentiation.
- **B.** Usually runs a more prolonged course than does osteosarcoma.
- **C.** May arise from a pre-existing benign cartilage tumour.
- **D.** Commonly arises in the pelvis or ribs.
- **E.** Commonly occurs under the age of 30 years.

25.8 **Rheumatoid arthritis:**
- **A.** Is usually associated with a negative test for rheumatoid factor during the active phase of the disease.
- **B.** Is associated with rheumatoid nodules in nearly all cases.
- **C.** May give rise to radial deviation of the fingers.
- **D.** Usually has microscopic appearances of villous hypertrophy of the synovium with inflammatory cells.
- **E.** Affects about 3% of the female population in Britain.

(Answers overleaf)

25.6 **A.** **True.** Type I collagen forms 90% of the matrix of bone and all types of osteogenesis imperfecta are characterised by abnormal synthesis of this type of collagen.

  B. **True.** The sclerae are often thinner than usual and appear blue due to the visibility of the choroid.

  C. **True.** In the lethal perinatal type of osteogenesis imperfecta multiple fractures occur in utero and may cause death before birth.

  D. **False.** Most types of osteogenesis imperfecta are transmitted by an autosomal dominant pattern of inheritance but the perinatal lethal type usually has an autosomal recessive pattern.

  E. **True.** This hearing loss is due to bony abnormalities of the inner and middle ear.

25.7 **A.** **False.** Chondrosarcomas show cartilagenous differentiation.

  B. **True.** Chondrosarcoma often recurs locally and may kill the patient by involvement of a vital structure. It does not metastasise as readily as osteosarcoma so the course of the disease is often more prolonged.

  C. **True.** About 10% of chondrosarcomas are thought to arise from pre-existing benign tumours of cartilage.

  D. **True.** Some 50% of chondrosarcomas arise in these sites.

  E. **False.** Chondrosarcomas are rare under the age of 30 years; most arise in subjects between 40 and 70 years of age.

25.8 **A.** **False.** Tests for rheumatoid factor are usually positive during the active phase of the disease.

  B. **False.** Subcutaneous nodules over pressure areas occur in about 20% of cases. They tend to occur in the more severely affected patients and to be associated with a worse prognosis.

  C. **False.** The fingers usually deviate in the ulnar direction with atrophy of the intrinsic muscles of the hand.

  D. **True.** There is marked villous hypertrophy of the synovium with aggregates of lymphocytes and a diffuse plasma cell infiltrate. In the early stages there may be fibrin deposition and many neutrophils.

  E. **True.** It also affects about 1% of the male population; only a small proportion of those affected become severely crippled.

26

Central and peripheral nervous systems

26.1 Central chromatolysis of a neurone:
- A. Is followed by regeneration in a neurone of the central nervous system.
- B. Is accompanied by a decrease in protein synthesis.
- C. Occurs 1–2 days after the severance of a neurone.
- D. Is characterised by disappearance of the Nissl granules, leaving a pale homogeneous cytoplasm.
- E. May occur as a response to certain viral infections.

26.2 The following are neuroglial cells:
- A. Oligodendrocytes.
- B. Microglia.
- C. Ependymal cells.
- D. Astrocytes.
- E. Neurones.

26.3 Raised intracranial pressure may produce:
- A. Diminished consciousness.
- B. Erosion of the posterior clinoid processes.
- C. Papilloedema.
- D. Lowered systolic blood pressure with a rapid pulse.
- E. Tonsillar herniation.

26.1 **A.** **False.** Neurones of the central nervous system are incapable of regeneration. Central chromatolysis may be followed by regeneration in peripheral nerves.

B. **False.** Central chromatolysis is accompanied by an increase in protein synthesis and so is thought to be an attempt at regeneration.

C. **False.** Central chromatolysis occurs 5–8 days after severance of a neurone.

D. **True.** This is the characteristic appearance which gives the process its name.

E. **True.** It may also occur in some vitamin B group deficiencies.

26.2 **A.** **True.** These cells have a neuroectodermal origin. They derive their name from the fact that they have a few short protoplasmic processes.

B. **False.** These cells belong to the monocyte–phagocyte system.

C. **True.** These cells have a neuroectodermal origin. They form a single layer of cells lining the ventricular system and central canal of the spinal cord.

D. **True.** These cells have a neuroectodermal origin. They form the principal supporting tissue of the central nervous system.

E. **False.** Neurones are not glial cells.

26.3 **A.** **True.** Raised intracranial pressure can produce diminished consciousness and eventually coma.

B. **True.** Chronically raised intracranial pressure may result in erosion of the posterior clinoid processes and other parts of the skull. The changes may be evident in radiographs of the skull.

C. **True.** Papilloedema is caused by compression of the retinal vein where it traverses the subarachnoid space in the optic sheath.

D. **False.** Raised intracranial pressure produces raised systolic blood pressure with a slow pulse rate.

E. **True.** Raised intracranial pressure can cause impaction of the cerebellar tonsils in the foramen magnum. This is especially likely to occur with space-occupying lesions below the tentorium.

26.4 **Hydrocephalus may occur in the following conditions:**
- **A.** Tuberculous meningitis.
- **B.** Tumours of the acoustic nerve.
- **C.** Intrauterine toxoplasmosis.
- **D.** Senile dementia.
- **E.** Arnold–Chiari malformation.

26.5 **Primary intracerebral haemorrhage:**
- **A.** Occurs most commonly in the region of the basal ganglia and the internal capsule.
- **B.** Occurs from micro-aneurysms on small perforating arteries.
- **C.** Is often caused by ruptured berry aneurysms.
- **D.** Shows characteristic Lewy bodies on microscopic examination.
- **E.** Is associated with hypertension.

26.6 **Astrocytomas:**
- **A.** If well differentiated, are often called glioblastomas.
- **B.** Usually have well-demarcated borders on microscopic examination.
- **C.** Arise from neurones.
- **D.** Are the commonest type of glioma.
- **E.** Rarely show cystic change.

(Answers overleaf)

26.4 **A.** **True.** Fibrous tissue formation may lead to obliteration of the subarachnoid space, particularly in the basal cisterns.
B. **True.** Tumours of the acoustic nerve may compress the aqueduct and the fourth ventricle, thus producing hydrocephalus.
C. **True.** Intrauterine toxoplasmosis can produce meningitis and ventriculitis which may lead to obliteration of the subarachnoid space or the aqueduct.
D. **True.** Generalised reduction in the amount of brain tissue in senile dementia may lead to symmetrical enlargement of the ventricles.
E. **True.** This congenital malformation prevents cerebrospinal fluid from re-entering the cranial cavity through the foramen magnum.

26.5 **A.** **True.** The basal ganglia and internal capsule are the commonest sites of primary intracerebral haemorrhage. Other fairly common sites include the pons and cerebellum.
B. **True.** These micro-aneurysms occur more commonly in hypertensive subjects.
C. **False.** Ruptured berry aneurysms cause subarachnoid haemorrhage; there may be some intracerebral extension of the resulting haematoma.
D. **False.** Lewy bodies are characteristically found in the substantia nigra of subjects with Parkinson's disease.
E. **True.** Due to increased numbers of micro-aneurysms and the increased likelihood of rupturing these.

26.6 **A.** **False.** Anaplastic (undifferentiated) astrocytomas are called glioblastomas.
B. **False.** Although, macroscopically, astrocytomas may appear to have well-differentiated borders, they are diffusely infiltrative when examined microscopically.
C. **False.** Astrocytomas arise from astrocytes which are derived from the neuroectoderm.
D. **True.** Astrocytomas are the commonest type of gliomas. The other relatively common types are oligodendrogliomas and ependymomas.
E. **False.** Cystic change is common in astrocytomas, particularly cerebellar astrocytomas in childhood.

26.7 Meningiomas:

A. Account for 15–20% of primary intracranial tumours.
B. Are thought to arise from the arachnoid granulations.
C. Are usually malignant.
D. Microscopically, often show psammoma bodies and whorl formation.
E. Are common in Lindau's disease.

26.8 von Recklinghausen's disease:

A. Features multiple neurofibromas along small nerve branches.
B. Is usually associated with multiple pigmented patches of skin.
C. Is not associated with mental retardation.
D. Is associated with an increased incidence of meningiomas and gliomas.
E. Is inherited in an autosomal recessive pattern.

26.9 The cerebrospinal fluid in chronic tuberculous meningitis:

A. Contains markedly increased numbers of neutrophil polymorphs.
B. May show acid-fast bacilli on Ziehl–Neelsen staining.
C. Usually appears blood-stained.
D. Usually has increased levels of glucose.
E. Is usually at a decreased pressure.

(Answers overleaf)

26.7 **A. True.** Meningiomas are the second commonest type of primary intracranial tumours after gliomas.
   B. True.
   C. False. Meningiomas are usually benign and can be removed by surgery with considerable success (they are a fairly common incidental finding at autopsy).
   D. True. These are the characteristic microscopic features of meningiomas.
   E. False. Haemangioblastomas are the tumours associated with Lindau's disease.

26.8 **A. True.** Neurofibromatosis is a synonym for von Recklinghausen's disease.
   B. True. 'Café au lait' spots are usually part of the syndrome.
   C. False. About 10% of cases have mental retardation and epilepsy due to a diffuse cortical dysgenesis.
   D. True. The reason for the increased incidence of meningiomas and gliomas is unclear.
   E. False. von Recklinghausen's disease is inherited by an autosomal dominant pattern of inheritance though, strangely, males are usually more severely affected than females.

26.9 **A. False.** Although a few neutrophils may be found at the start of tuberculous meningitis, the increase in cerebrospinal cellularity in the chronic infection is almost entirely due to mononuclear cells.
   B. True. Tubercle bacilli may be seen by direct staining methods but culture is a more sensitive method of detection.
   C. False. The cerebrospinal fluid is usually clear or slightly opalescent in tuberculous meningitis. Blood-stained cerebrospinal fluid may be due to subarachnoid haemorrhage or to passing the lumbar puncture needle through a spinal blood vessel.
   D. False. Glucose levels in the cerebrospinal fluid are usually lowered in tuberculous meningitis.
   E. False. The pressure of the cerebrospinal fluid is usually raised to as much as 300 mm of water.

26.10 In tabes dorsalis:
A. The Argyll Robertson phenomenon may be present.
B. There are often increased numbers of lymphocytes in the CSF.
C. There may be a neuropathic arthropathy.
D. There is pallor in the posterior columns of the spinal cord when stained by the Weigert–Pal method.
E. The posterior nerve roots entering the thoracic spinal cord are most commonly affected.

26.11 Acute necrotising encephalitis due to herpes simplex infection:
A. May be diagnosed by brain biopsy.
B. Is the commonest type of acute encephalitis in Europe.
C. Usually affects the frontal lobes most severely.
D. Rarely causes death.
E. Shows meningeal infiltration by lymphocytes and plasma cells.

26.12 Poliovirus:
A. Selectively attacks the motor neurone cells in the anterior horn of the spinal cord.
B. Is most readily isolated from the faeces of infected subjects.
C. Occurs in three different types.
D. Produces neurological signs in the majority of those infected.
E. Gains entry to the central nervous system across the blood–brain barrier.

(Answers overleaf)

26.10 A. True. In this phenomenon pupils contract normally during accommodation but not in response to light.

B. True. There are usually 50 or more lymphocytes per microlitre, and some macrophages.

C. True. The sensory neuropathy can lead to damage to the joints. Affected joints are sometimes called 'Charcot's joints'.

D. True. The Weigert–Pal method stains myelin blue, so the posterior columns will appear pale due to loss of myelinated fibres.

E. False. The lumbar enlargement of the spinal cord is the commonest site followed by the cervical enlargement.

26.11 A. True. Brain biopsy is the usual method of diagnosis in life but therapy (acyclovir) is often given without this definitive method of diagnosis.

B. True.

C. False. The temporal lobes are usually affected most severely. Memory problems are common in survivors.

D. False. Acute necrotising encephalitis is often rapidly fatal.

E. True. This is the typical histological picture.

26.12 A. True. The motor neurone cells in the anterior horn are selectively attacked, particularly in the lumbar and cervical enlargements.

B. True. Poliovirus is an enterovirus and gains entry to the body via the oral route. It is excreted in the faeces.

C. True. Vaccines must contain all three types to be effective, and must be given three times to allow full immune response to each type.

D. False. Most of those infected with poliovirus develop a mild febrile illness without neurological problems or have no symptoms at all.

E. True. After colonising the gut, the poliovirus gains entry to the blood stream and can then cross the blood–brain barrier into the central nervous system.

26.13 The cerebrospinal fluid in acute pyogenic meningitis:

   A. Is usually clear.

   B. Usually has an increased glucose level.

   C. Usually has a decreased protein level.

   D. May show bacteria on Gram staining.

   E. Contains markedly increased numbers of neutrophil polymorphs.

26.14 Multiple sclerosis:

   A. Shows patchy demyelination irregularly distributed in the brain and spinal cord.

   B. Usually starts after the age of 50 years.

   C. Usually follows a regular, progressive course.

   D. May show an increase in protein concentration of the cerebrospinal fluid with an oligoclonal pattern.

   E. Often presents as an acute unilateral optic neuritis.

26.15 Senile dementia of Alzheimer's type:

   A. Is commoner in males than in females.

   B. Shows reduced numbers of argyrophilic plaques when examined microscopically.

   C. Often shows primary hydrocephalus.

   D. Usually shows widespread cortical atrophy.

   E. Is caused by multiple cerebral infarcts.

(Answers overleaf)

26.13 A. False. The cerebrospinal fluid in acute pyogenic
   meningitis is usually turbid or frankly purulent.
   B. False. Glucose is absent or greatly reduced.
   C. False. Protein is usually raised in the cerebrospinal fluid
   in acute pyogenic meningitis.
   D. True. The type of bacteria must be confirmed by culture.
   E. True. There may be as many as 500–5000 neutrophils
   per microlitre of cerebrospinal fluid in acute pyogenic
   meningitis. Mononuclear inflammatory cells (lymphocytes
   and monocytes) appear later in the infection.

26.14 A. True. These areas of demyelination are often called
   'plaques'.
   B. False. Multiple sclerosis usually starts in early adulthood.
   C. False. The characteristic course of multiple sclerosis is
   episodic with acute attacks occurring at irregular intervals.
   D. True. Lymphocyte numbers may also be increased.
   E. True. This common presenting symptom often
   progresses to some degree of optic atrophy.

26.15 A. False. It is found twice as commonly in females than in
   males.
   B. False. The characteristic histological feature of
   Alzheimer's disease is vastly increased numbers of
   argyrophilic plaques in the cortical grey matter. Other
   features include neurofibrillary tangles, loss of neurones
   and reactive gliosis.
   C. False. Dilation of the ventricular system occurs but this is
   secondary to loss of cortical tissue.
   D. True. The atrophy is usually most conspicuous at the
   frontal and temporal poles.
   E. False. Senile dementia of Alzheimer's type is a primary
   dementia for which no cause has yet been found.
   Dementia can occur after multiple cerebral infarcts.

26.16 Chronic subdural haematoma:
  A. Is rare in the young and old.
  B. Is always associated with a history of head injury.
  C. Rarely produces symptoms.
  D. Is caused by arterial bleeding.
  E. Is rarely bilateral.

26.17 Retinoblastoma:
  A. Has a positive association with deletion of the long arm of chromosome 13.
  B. Has a 5-year survival rate of about 90%.
  C. Is familial in 80% of cases.
  D. Shows a primitive neuroectodermal pattern of differentiation.
  E. Often produces distant metastases.

26.18 Chronic otitis media may produce the following complications:
  A. Tympanic perforation.
  B. Aural polyps.
  C. Cholesteatomas.
  D. Disarticulation of the ossicles.
  E. Paragangliomas.

26.19 Duchenne-type muscular dystrophy:
  A. Usually presents in the third decade of life.
  B. Has an autosomal dominant pattern of inheritance.
  C. Arises as a result of spontaneous mutation in one-third of cases.
  D. Occurs in about 1 in 350 live-born males.
  E. Features central nuclei in muscle fibres.

(Answers overleaf)

26.16 A. False. The young and old are most commonly affected by chronic subdural haematomas.

B. False. There may be no history of head injury since very trivial injury can lead to a subdural haematoma in the elderly.

C. False. Unilateral neurological symptoms or confusion mimicking senile dementia are common.

D. False. Bleeding originates from the cortical bridging veins.

E. False. Bilaterality of subdural haematomas is quite common.

26.17 A. True. This deletion always involves a specific site and is of great interest to those investigating carcinogenesis because it may involve deletion of an anti-oncogene.

B. True. Enucleation of the eye and radiotherapy produces a high rate of survival.

C. False. It is familial in 10–15% of cases.

D. True. This pattern is characterised by small dark cells, some arranged in a rosette pattern.

E. False. Although retinoblastoma may spread along the optic nerve or invade through the sclera it rarely produces distant metastases.

26.18 A. True.

B. True. These polyps are composed of granulation tissue.

C. True. These are accumulations of keratotic debris which occur after squamous epithelium has spread into the middle ear after tympanic perforation.

D. True. This may lead to a conductive hearing loss.

E. False. These are tumours arising from the chemoreceptor cells in glomus jugulare and are not a complication of chronic otitis media.

26.19 A. False. Duchenne-type muscular dystrophy presents in childhood.

B. False. It has an X-linked recessive pattern of inheritance.

C. True. Two-thirds arise from mothers who are carrying the defective gene on one of their X-chromosomes.

D. False. It occurs in about 1 in 3000–5000 live-born males.

E. True. Other histological features include contraction bands, macrophages and fibre splitting.

26.20 Dermatomyositis:

   A. Is commoner in males than in females.

   B. Usually affects distal muscles early in the course of the disease.

   C. Classically produces heliotrope discolouration of the upper eyelids.

   D. Often affects the ocular muscles.

   E. Histologically shows fragmentation of the sarcoplasm.

26.21 Myasthenia gravis:

   A. Is more common in males than in females.

   B. Has a positive association with thymomas.

   C. Is associated with organ-specific autoimmune diseases.

   D. Often affects the external ocular muscles.

   E. Is usually associated with antibodies to acetylcholine receptors.

26.22 Parkinson's disease:

   A. Causes deafness.

   B. Usually presents in the third decade of life.

   C. Is characterised histologically by Lewy bodies.

   D. Produces bradykinesia.

   E. Is an autosomal recessive disorder.

(Answers overleaf)

26.20 **A.** **False.** Dermatomyositis is twice as common in females as it is in males.
  B. **False.** The myopathy which accompanies dermatomyositis affects the proximal muscles before the distal muscles.
  C. **True.** This is the dramatic appearance which dermatomyositis can produce.
  D. **False.** Dermatomyositis very rarely affects the ocular muscles. This provides a striking contrast with myasthenia gravis.
  E. **True.** Later in the disease, fibrosis and muscular atrophy may be the predominant features.

26.21 **A.** **False.** Myasthenia gravis is more common in women than in men.
  B. **True.** Most cases of myasthenia gravis are associated with thymic hyperplasia but many cases which develop in middle age are associated with thymomas.
  C. **True.** Diseases such as Hashimoto's thyroiditis are associated with myasthenia gravis.
  D. **True.** These muscles are usually some of the first to be affected. Ptosis and blurred vision are common presenting symptoms.
  E. **True.** Over 90% of subjects with myasthenia gravis have antibodies to the acetylcholine receptor of skeletal muscle.

26.22 **A.** **False.** Deafness is a feature of Friedreich's ataxia, which is another neurodegenerative disorder.
  B. **False.** Symptoms usually become manifest in the fifth and sixth decades of life.
  C. **True.** These inclusions are found in dopaminergic neurones in the substantia nigra and locus caeruleus.
  D. **True.** The other clinical features are rigidity and tremor.
  E. **False.** There is no described inherited element to Parkinson's disease. Friedreich's ataxia has an autosomal recessive mode of inheritance.

26.23 Huntington's chorea:

  A. Has an X-linked pattern of inheritance.
  B. Is characterised by atrophy of the caudate nucleus and putamen.
  C. Usually presents in the second decade of life.
  D. May be manifest as a personality change with depression.
  E. Is associated with reduced levels of choline acetyltransferase in the basal ganglia.

26.24 The following pathologies may occur in the CNS of those infected by the human immunodeficiency virus:

  A. Cytomegalovirus infection.
  B. Primary cerebral lymphoma.
  C. Toxoplasmosis.
  D. Dementia.
  E. Fungal infection.

26.25 Motor neurone disease:

  A. Occurs more often in females than males.
  B. Usually presents before the age of 20 years.
  C. May involve the cranial nerve motor nuclei.
  D. Usually causes death due to respiratory failure.
  E. In the familial form is associated with a mutation in the superoxide dismutase gene on chromosome 21q.

(Answers overleaf)

26.23 A. False. Huntington's chorea has an autosomal dominant pattern of inheritance.
B. True. Histologically these areas show a loss of small neurones.
C. False. The disease usually becomes apparent in the fifth decade of life.
D. True. Later in the disease process movement disorders, such as choreiform movements, appear.
E. True. This may be secondary to the neuronal loss.

26.24 A. True. Other opportunistic viral infections include the papovaviruses.
B. True.
C. True. Another opportunistic infection.
D. True. A dementia caused by the HIV virus may occur, even in the absence of full-blown AIDS.
E. True. Fungi are common opportunistic infective agents in AIDS.

26.25 A. False. Motor neurone disease occurs more frequently in males than females.
B. False. Presentation is usually after the age of 50 years.
C. True. This produces the progressive bulbar palsy variant of the disease with weakness of the tongue, palate and pharyngeal muscles.
D. True. This is the usual cause of death. Patients may have their lives prolonged by mechanical ventilation; this has led to many ethical dilemmas which have led to court cases in the United States.
E. True. The familial form is only identified in about 5% of cases of motor neurone disease.

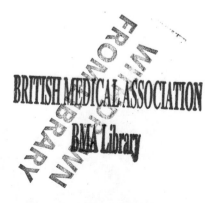